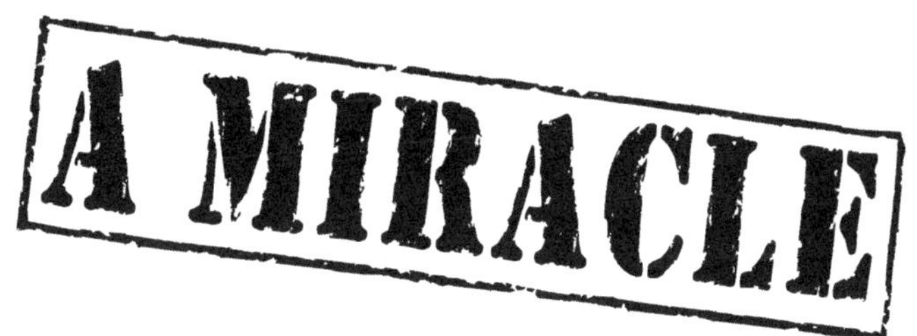

Attie De Vries

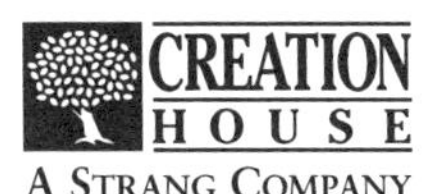

A Miracle by Attie De Vries
Published by Creation House
A Strang Company
600 Rinehart Road
Lake Mary, Florida 32746
www.creationhouse.com

Cover design by Amanda Potter

Library of Congress Control Number: 2007940831
International Standard Book Number: 978-1-59979-311-5

First Edition

08 09 10 11 12 — 987654321
Printed in the United States of America

This book is lovingly dedicated to our mother and grandma, Janke van der Veen. She prayed faithfully for all of us and always believed that with the Lord all things are possible

CONTENTS

Then the Lord answered me and said, record the vision and inscribe it on tablets, that the one who reads it may run. "For the vision is yet for the appointed time; it hastens toward the goal, and it will not fail. Though it tarries, wait for it; for it will certainly come, it will not delay."

—Habakkuk 2:2–3, NASB

INTRODUCTION

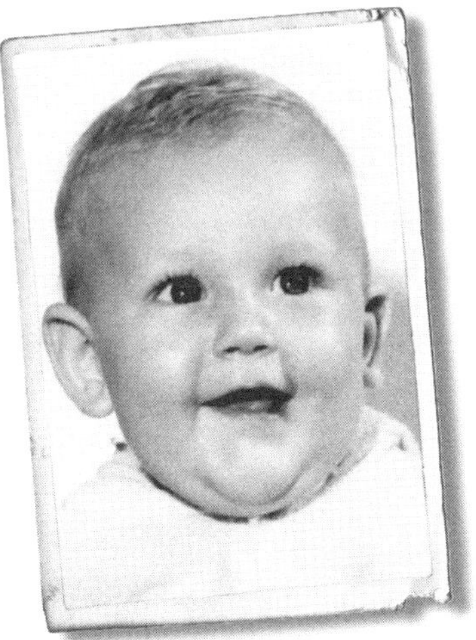

Baby Simon

He is a real boy, Mrs. De Vries!" the nurse standing at my bedside told me as she handed me our first son, Simon. He was a beautiful little boy with blond hair and blue eyes. As I looked at his face for the first time, it was as if I had known him all my life. Little did I realize that one day I would look back at that moment and know there was something very special about that day—God was there!

This is the story of one family and how a tragedy became a blessing.

Several years ago, our son Simon was diagnosed with an incurable disease called scleroderma, a disease of uncontrolled tissue growth in the skin and internal organs. God turned around what seemed to us an impossible situation and healed Simon.

This book deals with some of the fears and frustrations we had, but even more, it describes how fighting the disease brought us to a greater awareness of God. As a result of Simon's illness, we turned to the Lord for all the answers.

We learned how dependent we are on the Lord for everything we need. In the midst of our struggle, God even supplied the necessary faith the very moment when we needed it. Some of the things we learned through these experiences became keys that unlocked life-changing power in our lives and in the life of Simon as God began to heal him.

With God, everything is possible if we are surrendered to His will. No matter what we face in life, God is the answer!

It is my prayer that in sharing our story with you, the Lord will bless and touch you. Hopefully you will be able to say, "All things work together for good to them that love God, to them who are the called according to his purpose" (Rom. 8:28, KJV).

Jesus replied, "Love the Lord Your God with all of your heart, soul, and mind."

—Matthew 23:37, TLB

1

COMING TO AMERICA

I WAS BORN IN the Netherlands, in Friesland, a tiny speck on the world map. If you look at the map of Europe, take your magnifying glass and you will see Holland on the left of the map, next to Belgium and Germany. If you look even closer up in the northern part of Holland, you will see Friesland, an island by itself, so to speak. I was born in Leeuwarden, which is the capitol of Friesland. If you drive from the airport, Schiphol, to Alkmaar and then to Den Helder, you go over a big dike in the middle of the sea, called the Afsluit dike. Then you arrive at the town of Leeuwarden. It has an atmosphere of its own, back in time.

My mother was born in Opeinde, by Drachten. My dad was born in Leeuwarden. They came from two different worlds. Mom came from a Christian home, and Dad from a non-Christian home. Mom was raised on a farm, and Dad was raised in the city. Mom could not wait to go to the big city, Leeuwarden, which is where she met my dad.

My grandfather was opposed to Mom marrying my father, but she did marry Dad. Three years after I was born, the war broke out. I remember airplanes flying over our home in the middle of the night. On the radio, we heard that the Germans had invaded Holland and we were at war.

My grandfather made a great impression on me as a little girl. He knew the Lord. We spent a lot of time at our grandparents' home. We called them Pake and Beppe. They had a couple of acres of land, so we city kids could play to our hearts' content out in the field. At night, we sat around the fire. My grandfather talked about God, what was going on in the world, and the war.

"There was a time in my life," he said, "I was drinking too much." He told us God spoke to him as he drove his milk wagon down the street in Opeinde. The Lord said to him, "Jan, I do not want you to drink anymore." So, my grandfather came home, poured the liquor down the drain, and never touched another drop again. The year must have been 1916 or so.

Mom and Dad divorced when I was seven years old. I, being the oldest, took on a lot of the responsibilities. Mom did not go to church, but she did believe there was a God and sent all of us children to a Christian school where I heard the gospel, how Jesus died for our sins on the cross. At the age of seven, I gave my heart to the Lord at the Salvation Army. For about three years I prayed for my mother every night, until one Sunday evening a neighbor took Mom to the Salvation Army.

My mother said later that evening that it was the first time she heard the good news that God loved her. And as she has said so many times since, "Then there is at least One that loves me." She came forward, knelt, and accepted the Lord. She became a new person in Christ, "Old things have passed away; behold, all things have become new" (2 Cor. 5:17).

From then on we had a different home life. We all went to church every Sunday. I thank the Lord for saving my mother that day.

In 1952, I met my husband, Simen, at a ballroom dance on a Saturday evening. As my husband explained later, he saw two cute girls walking in front of him. He said to his friend, "Wherever those two are going, we go. You take the red-haired girl and I'll take the dark-haired girl," which happened to be me. I was fifteen and Simen was eighteen.

We discovered that we lived around the corner from each other. As I found out later, Simen had big plans for the future. He wanted to go to America, and he asked me how I felt about that. Well, I had mixed emotions about it. "What about my family?" I wondered to myself. It was not an easy decision to make; but then, I did not have to make it anytime soon. We were so young and Simen had to go into the Dutch Air Force for two years when I met him. A lot can change in that time. Or so I thought.

Simen and I went steady for four years before he immigrated to America. I followed one year later with all the excitement one feels when one is twenty years old, going overseas to a land that promises a glorious future. Life was full of adventure. Four weeks after I arrived in America, we married in a Dutch Christian Reformed service at the YMCA in Pasadena, California. The pastor was Frank De Jong, who started a Dutch-speaking church there.

We had always dreamed of having a large family one day, maybe ten children. So when we found out that we were going to have our first child, we were overjoyed! I remember it so well. Simen came home from work announcing, "At [that was his nickname for me], how would you like to go camping?"

"Camping," I asked. "Where?"

"Yosemite National Park," he said. "My co-worker said it is a beautiful place to camp."

"But, Simen, I don't feel so good." We thought I had a flu bug.

"Yeah, but in four weeks you'll feel better," Simen said. "How long can this last, right?"

Wrong. Four weeks later I was still sick, but we went anyway. I found out that Yosemite National Park really is a beautiful place to go camping. You can ride your bike in the woods or hike to the waterfalls. Or you can sit under a tree and read a book and dream, which I preferred because I still felt sick.

Camping next to us was a big family from New York. The mother had seen me throwing up. Suspecting something, she came over and talked to me. I was lying down in the tent. She took my husband aside and said, "I believe your wife is pregnant." Simen came back in the tent and told me what our neighbor had said.

"Me, pregnant? Oh, I hope so!" That evening we sat around the campfire discussing the possibility of my being pregnant. "Oh, please, God, give us a baby!" I prayed.

We decided to go home early to see a doctor and to find out if it was true. Now, you have to understand that Yosemite National Park is no picnic for a pregnant lady. There are too many winding roads. Descending the mountains, we had to stop the car several times so I could get sick in the gardenias by the side of the road.

After the visit to the doctor, we were thrilled when we heard the good news, "You were not carsick, Mrs. De Vries. You are going to have a baby!" We had waited for this for months, and yet it took us by surprise. What a blessing! We could not wait to tell our family. I called my mother in Holland to tell her that she was going to be a grandmother for the first time.

She also had some news to share. They had just received a letter from the Dutch Immigration Service stating that they could immigrate to the United States. We were so glad—a baby and being reunited with my family!

Mom, my two brothers, and my sister Tina arrived at Christmastime. First, they went from Holland by boat to New York. Then they took a bus to Los Angeles, arriving just in time for Christmas. We were all together as a family, awaiting the birth of our first child and grandchild.

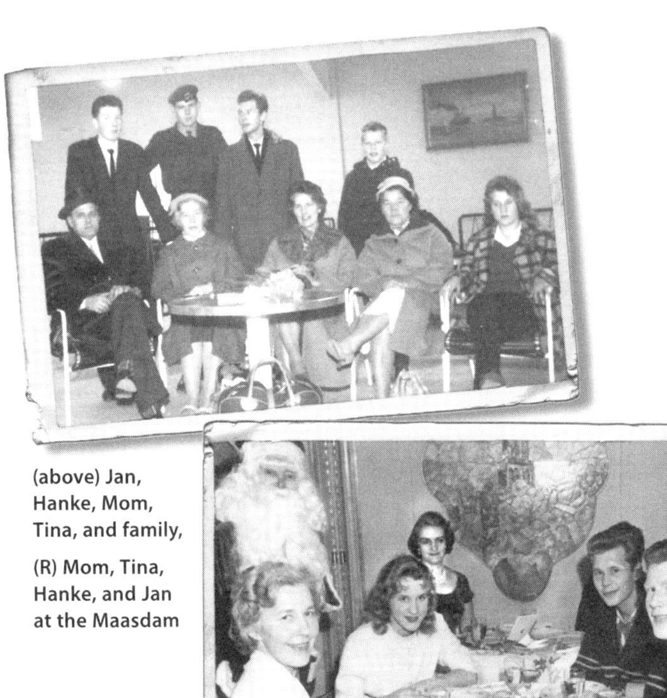

(above) Jan, Hanke, Mom, Tina, and family,

(R) Mom, Tina, Hanke, and Jan at the Maasdam

Jacqueline was born at six o'clock on a Thursday morning. She had big blue eyes and lots of dark hair, with a sparkling personality to match. She has been a blessing ever since.

Three years later I was pregnant again and told my husband it would be a boy. We were going to have a son! Some time later, I came to realize how very much Simen wanted a son. We were at a fabric store to purchase material for the bassinet I was going to make. I hesitated on the color. I wanted blue for a boy, but instead was going to take yellow, just in case it was a girl. My husband looked at me in amazement. "You said it was going to be a boy!"

"All right," I said, "I'll take the blue." The sales girl smiled at Simen's comment.

Sure enough, six weeks later our son Simon was born. Two years later, the Lord blessed us with another son, Michael. We were overjoyed in the delivery room when the doctor announced, "You have another little boy, Mrs. De Vries! Two boys—how blessed can you be!" the doctor said. Our son Michael had big green eyes and blond hair.

One and a half years later, our second daughter, Yvonne, was born. "A beautiful girl, dark hair and green eyes, just like a little China doll," the doctor exclaimed.

We thanked the Lord for giving them to us. I remember each time we baptized them at our church. To us it was a special occasion of promising the Lord to bring them up right. But the cares of daily living, being so busy, and wanting things, took me further away from the Lord.

It's not that the Lord does not want us to have things, but if those things become number one in your life, then they are idols. An idol is anything that stands between us and God—money, material things, or pleasure. "For where your treasure is, there your heart will be also" (Matt. 6:21). I still went to church and each time promised to do better, start a new week, read my Bible, pray, and spend time with God. But tomorrow was always another day, with more things to do and more concerns to distract.

There is a verse in Isaiah that explains what we go through so well:

> Is anyone thirsty? Come and drink—even if you have no money!... Why spend your money on food that doesn't give you strength? Why pay for groceries that do you no good? Listen and I'll tell you where to get good food that fattens up the soul!
>
> —Isaiah 55:1–2, TLB

This means, are you getting out of life what you want? Are you happy? Do "things" satisfy you? Do you have peace in your home? How is the relationship between you and your children? Well, Isaiah says that we can have this by coming to God to know Him, the Giver of life!

One Sunday morning our pastor quoted a scripture that touched me deeply, "You shall love the LORD your God with all your heart, with all your soul, and with all your mind.... You shall love your neighbor as yourself" (Matt. 22:37, 39). That week I had to think about the sermon's verse. "It is a difficult verse," I thought. "How can I love God, whom I have never seen? What about my neighbors? They are nice people, but do I love them? No, they are just nice people. What about God? How do I love God?" I pondered. This verse stayed with me. That day my relationship with God was irrevocably challenged.

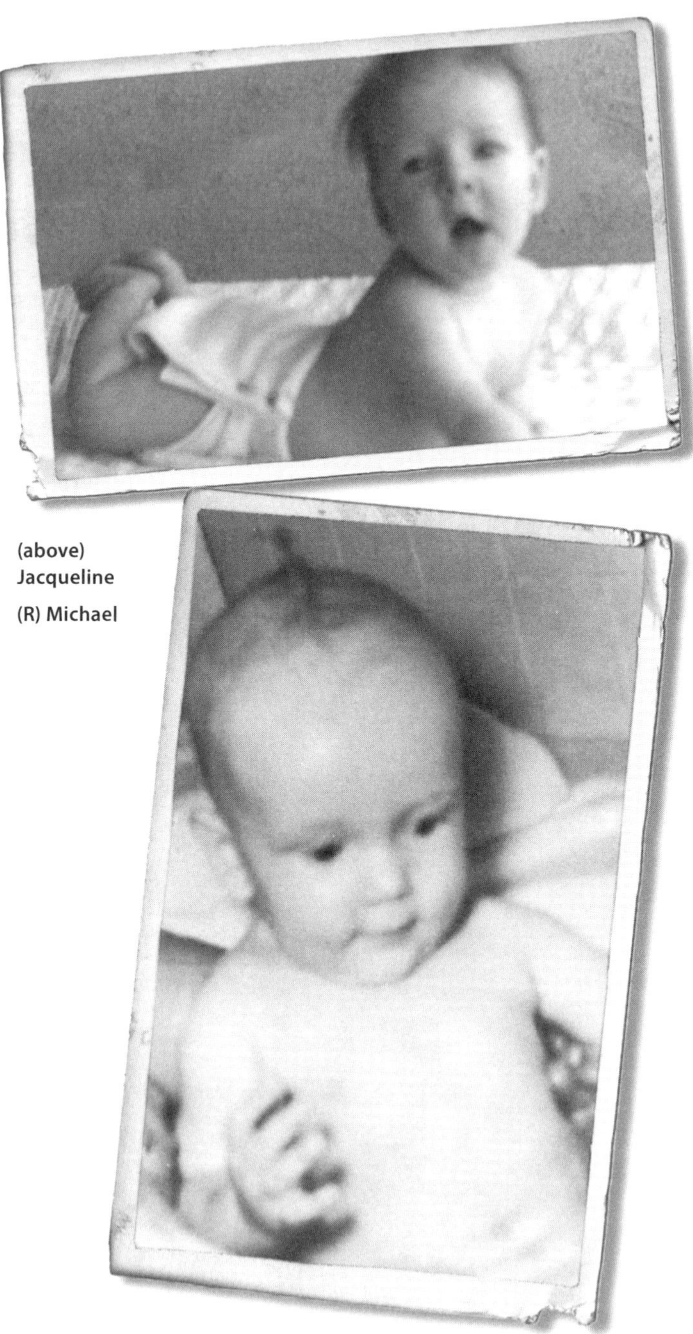

(above) Jacqueline

(R) Michael

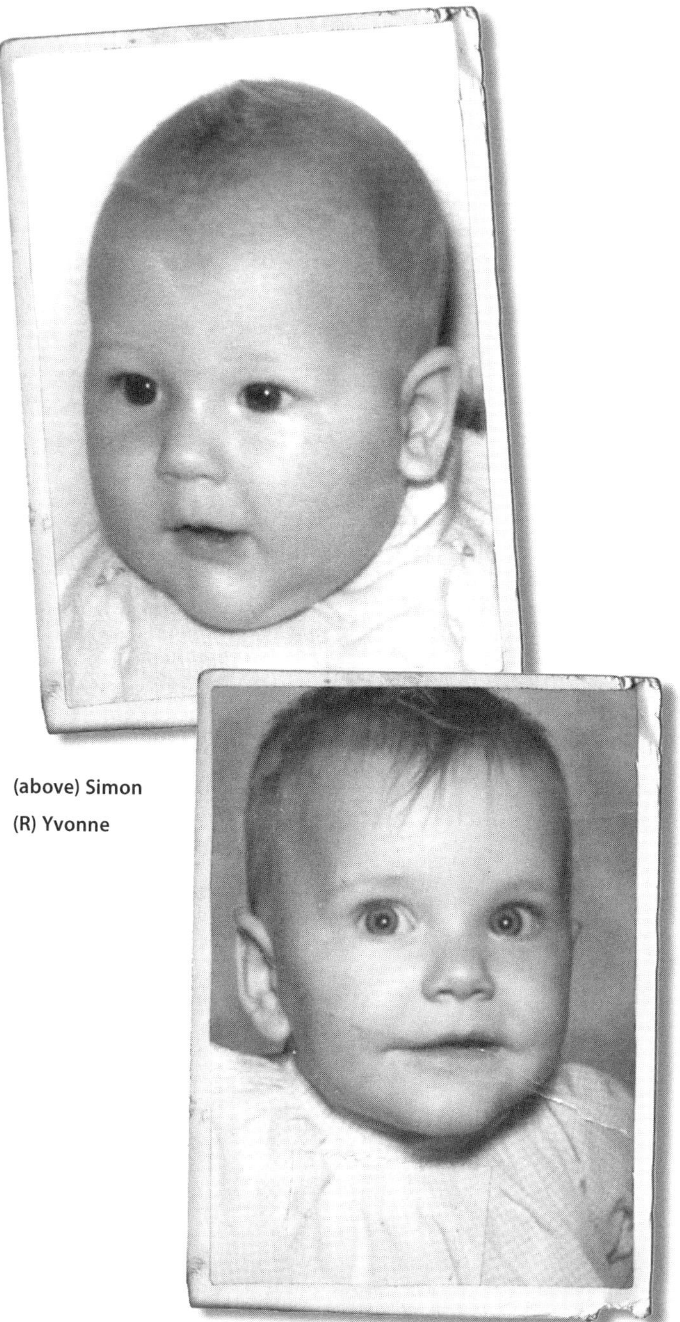

(above) Simon
(R) Yvonne

And which of you by being anxious can add a single cubit to his life's span?

—Matthew 6:27, NASB

2

DIAGNOSIS: SCLERODERMA

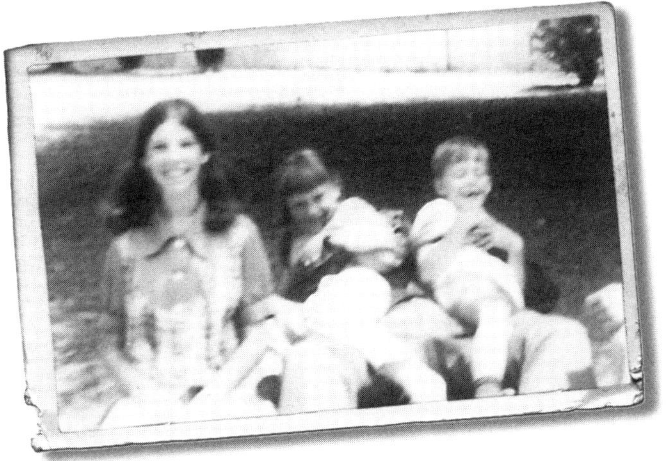

Jacqueline, Yvonne, and Michael playing with Simen

It was a beautiful, sunny day. The wind was slowly moving the leaves of our big Alder tree. Big gulps of sunlight came moving through the open windows. It was a peaceful afternoon. The only sound you could hear was the laughter of our children playing on the front lawn.

As I got up from where I was sitting, slowly walking toward the front window, I heard a loud bang behind me. Turning around, I looked directly at the face of our five-year-old son,

Simon, who had just stormed into the house, slamming the front door behind him.

"Mom, can you wash my hands? They're dirty." His smiling face looked up at me.

"Sure," I said, not realizing the painful discovery I was about to make. While washing his hands that afternoon, I noticed something strange. Simon was unable to turn them. Not expecting this, I said, "Sweetheart, what happened? Does it hurt when I turn your hands?"

"No, Mom," he said, "they don't hurt." And with that he ran outside to play.

"This is puzzling," I thought. The prior month, Simon had pain in his left ankle. We had an X-ray taken, but it revealed nothing. The doctor diagnosed it as a possible sprained muscle.

However, that afternoon I became alarmed. "Could there be a connection?" I wondered. "First his left ankle and now his hands?" I thought. As the children were playing outside, I began to plan what to do next. A feeling of fear began to gnaw at me. "Something is drastically wrong here," I thought. The next day I made an appointment to see our doctor, hoping there was an easy explanation for these symptoms.

As I examined Simon more carefully that evening, I became even more alarmed. Both of his arms were very stiff, and his ankle was still bothering him. The doctor had explained to me that a sprained muscle could take up to eight weeks to heal, and that was only two weeks ago. The next day the doctor examined Simon carefully.

"When did these symptoms first appear?" he asked. "What did you first notice?"

As I was answering the doctors' questions, my thoughts went to, "God, please let Simon be all right. He just has to be."

After the doctor finished asking all the routine questions, he examined Simon again. "Simon, make a fist with your hand," he said. Then, with some gravity in his voice, looking at me, he said, "Simon, squeeze your mom's hand." As he did, I knew something was wrong. Simon was not able to get a firm grip with his hands. A quiet panic began to arise within me. Not only was there something wrong with his foot, there was something wrong with his wrists and his hands, too.

"Oh, God," I prayed, "I hope there is nothing else wrong!"

"Simon, can you sit on the floor for me?" The doctor asked. Simon did this awkwardly.

"Now, I want you to get up for me," I heard the doctor say. Simon struggled to get up. I saw that he was having a very difficult time accomplishing a task as simple as this. "We better have him checked in at children's hospital for more tests," the doctor finally told me. "It could be a number of things."

"What do you suspect?" I said, almost afraid to ask.

"Well, it could be one of the collagen diseases," he answered. With that, he explained that the collagen diseases are a family of illnesses such as rheumatoid arthritis, lupus, poly arthritis, and scleroderma. At that point, he could not be sure until further tests were done.

Driving home, I felt so many conflicting emotions. This had slowly crept up on all of us. We knew that Simon had difficulty getting up, but we had attributed that to the pain in his ankle. I tried desperately to calm the fear I felt inside. "Maybe it is not that bad," I reasoned. "Even if it is something serious, I am sure the doctor can help us," I concluded. I was smiling on the outside, but inside I was crying. "Strange," I thought, "how life can change in forty-eight hours."

Simen was waiting for us when we came home. "Well," he said, "did you find out anything?" He looked at me hopefully. I explained to him what the doctor had shared with me, and that he was going to make an appointment for us at the children's hospital in Los Angeles. We did not know what to say or think. We hoped that there would be a simple explanation or even a medical treatment to help his symptoms and that everything would turn out all right. We did not know what to expect.

Our next appointment was with a doctor who dealt with muscular diseases. He put Simon through some of the same tests as the first doctor. After he was finished, he asked me to step outside so he could check Simon's nerve impulses throughout his body. When I sat outside that room, I heard the cries of our little son. I could not help but feel powerless. After thirty minutes of testing, the doctor came and asked me to step back into the room.

"Can you tell me what is wrong?" I asked. "What are the results of the test?"

"No," he said. "We have to wait until all the test results are in. In the meantime, I want you to see another doctor. I will set up an appointment for you," he said. There seemed to be no clear answer.

Soon there were more tests, more biopsies, and more doctors. Simon had to be hospitalized for days and weeks at a time. It seemed endless, waiting for the results of all the tests, talking to doctors, waiting in the hospital. I used to think that you just went to the doctor, found out what was wrong or not wrong, and take it from there. I found out that life is not that clear-cut. There are no instant answers. Life had become very complicated.

After weeks of uncertainty, the doctor called us. His diagnosis was rheumatoid arthritis. "However," he cautioned, "we cannot be totally sure until all the results are in."

I knew what rheumatoid arthritis was, and I also knew that it was a very painful and crippling disease. "At least," I thought, "it is not a more serious disease." So, we tried to accept it and make the best of it.

During all of this time, we never asked the Lord to heal Simon. I knew it would take a miracle, and miracles only took place during the apostolic age, or so I thought. Therefore, I could not expect God to perform a miracle during the twentieth century.

The following Sunday morning, sitting in church, I looked around at all the familiar faces I had known for so long. "Are there more people who feel like I do, so far away from the Lord?" I wondered. It scared me to think that I had come to the place of asking, "Does God really know me?" Or worse yet, "Do I believe there is a God?" It was a wake-up call to say the least.

I was close to the Lord after I had accepted Him as my personal Savior at the young age of seven. But in my teen years I changed. I began to question my beliefs, going my own way, not putting the Lord in the center of my life, and slowly drifting away from Him to the ultimate place of questioning, "Is there a God?" I had no firm foundation to stand on. It was indeed a lonely place to be.

This was a whole different life, a life I was not prepared for, a life where there was so much sorrow and pain and worry. People like me try to cope with what life hands them. How can you prepare? You take health for granted, and you take for granted that your children are healthy. All of those little things that we, as parents, can fret about are no longer important when you enter the hospital wing where children are being treated for all kinds of diseases.

Many times, walking through the corridor at the hospital with Simon holding my hand, I thought about how life had changed. "There are no guarantees in life," I reminded myself. Looking at his face as he walked next to me, I would have given my life so that he could be healed. I was determined to make life pleasant for him; life had to go on. Yet, there was that nagging question. Since the doctor was not absolutely certain of his diagnosis, what if Simon didn't have rheumatoid arthritis?

In the meantime, Simon began to experience more and more symptoms in his muscles. He became weaker throughout his body. There were nights that he was in extreme pain due to spasms in his muscles. The only thing we could do to relieve the pain was to give Simon a painkiller, a hot bath, and massage his muscles. After sleeping for a while, Simon would wake up with painful stiffness throughout his body. All of the muscles in his arms and legs went into spasms, so a warm bath would help for a while until he fell asleep, only to wake up with the same problem again. This repeated itself quite a few times during the night. He did not have this problem as acutely during the day since his daily activity kept his joints moving somewhat. At times like these, my husband and I felt so helpless. To hear our son cry out in pain was devastating to both of us.

After about one year of this, the doctor called, wanting us to come in. The rest of the test results were in and he wanted to go over them with us. When he entered the room and sat down, I knew the news was not going to be good. "Simon does not have rheumatoid arthritis, as we had first suspected," he said. "He has scleroderma."

I didn't say anything for a moment. Finally, I said, "I know." The doctor and I had talked about this disease. We had suspected it, because two months prior to this we had noticed liver-colored spots on Simon's elbows and legs and a general hardening of his skin over these areas, which is typical in scleroderma.

The word *scleroderma* means "hard skin." The disease may affect all of the vital organs of the body, including the heart, liver, kidney, lungs, and the skin tissue. The covering of all of these organs will get progressively harder and less pliable because the body produces too much of a protein called collagen, resulting in intense pain in every area of the body. There is no cure for this disease. It is extremely painful and eventually fatal. There are about 400,000 Americans suffering from scleroderma.[1]

This was not what I had hoped for. As we drove home, I was extremely upset.

"Mom, can we stop for a hamburger?" Simon asked. "I am so hungry!"

Looking at his little face next to me, I said, "Sure, honey!"

"How can I ever tell him, or even share this with him?" I wondered. "Life is so simple at his age." All he was thinking about was a hamburger.

When we came home, Simon's dad opened the door and our eyes met. There was sadness; my husband knew. He put his arms around me and whispered, "The news isn't good, is it, At?"

I nodded my head and cried. "Simon has scleroderma," was all I could say. Until that morning, we had still clung to some hope, but now all hope was gone. There was nothing but despair—utter despair! I felt keenly the words of King Solomon, "In my opinion, nothing is worthwhile; everything is futile. For what does a man get for all his hard work?" (Eccl. 1:2–3, TLB). There was no hope left in our lives that day.

As the disease progressed, Simon developed an infection in his hips that caused extreme pain. As a result, he was unable to walk for days at a time. I was desperate by this time, and occasionally waves of panic overwhelmed me. At times it seemed more than I could bear.

One day my mom came over, and as I was making a cup of tea for us, fear struck. I looked at my mother and said, "Things aren't going so good with Simon." I guess the reality of it all just dawned on me at that moment. Mom and I looked at each other and we cried. It was in moments like that when I vented my emotions. I knew my mother was praying for us,

---

1. Henry Scammell, *Scleroderma* (New York: M. Evans and Co., 1998). See also "Scleroderma Risk Factors," *The New York Times* online, http://health.nytimes.com/health/guides/disease/scleroderma/risk-factors.html (accessed Nov. 27, 2007).

and many times she would say, "Attie, ask the Lord to help you. He can heal Simon!"

"The doctor said there is no cure, Mom," I said. My mother did not take no for an answer. She was convinced that the Lord could heal Simon, but I argued, "Healing is not for this age, Mom. That only took place in New Testament times."

"Well, I don't know about that," Mom said. "I have seen people being healed at a miracle service on TV." I did not say anything. What could I say? I just did not know how the Lord could help us. My question was, "Does God even know about us?"

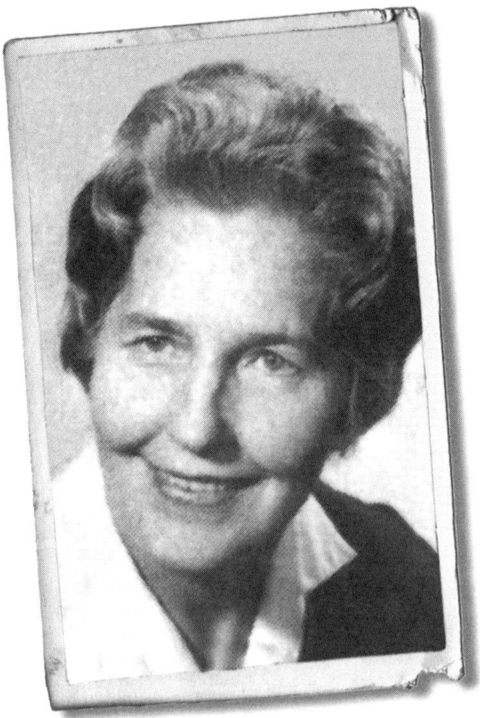

Oma, Jane

But all these things that I once thought very worthwhile—now I've thrown them all away so that I can put my trust and hope in Christ alone. Yes, everything else is worthless when compared with the priceless gain of knowing Christ Jesus my Lord. I have put aside all else, counting it worth less than nothing in order that I can have Christ.

—Philippians 3:7–8, NASB

3

GOD, I WANT TO KNOW YOU

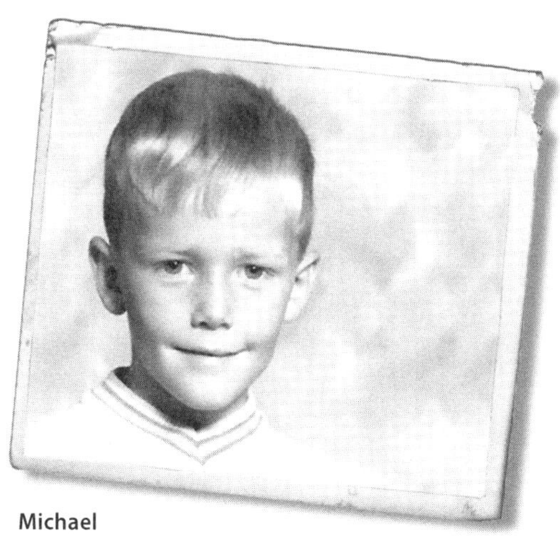

Michael

"MOM, ARE YOU getting up? It's seven o'clock!"

I recognized Michael's voice, calling me as he did every morning. I jumped out of bed. The De Vries house was full of life. One quick look at the clock told me it was time to make breakfast. Hurriedly, I got dressed. It was a beautiful, sunny morning. Walking into the kitchen, I was greeted by four little faces looking at me with expectation.

"Mom, can you make pancakes? Can you make hot cereal?"

"Pancakes it will be today," I said, and with this, my eyes caught sight of Simon sitting on the sofa. "Simon, don't you have to get dressed?"

"Yes, Mom, but I can't put on my socks!" His face was serious. His hands had become increasingly painful for him. I wanted to help him, but as the physical therapist had explained to me, Simon needed to dress himself. It was good exercise for him, but seeing him in such distress was difficult for me.

After we finished breakfast, I drove our children to school. As I observed them getting out of the car, full of life and energy, I looked at Simon next to me, who had to crawl out of the car. By this time, he was unable to open or close the door. Many times our five-year-old son Michael would get out of the car first so that he could help Simon. Those were moments mixed with delight and pain at seeing our children helping one another.

As I came home that day in deep despair, I walked into the kitchen and, without thinking, turned on the radio. My thoughts were elsewhere that morning. "What was life all about? What happened to all those dreams I had of a nice home filled with happy, healthy children?" I pondered. "Simon is not healthy. He is in a lot of pain, and there is nothing I, or anyone else, can do for him," I complained.

It was at that exact moment that I allowed myself to really look at my life, and at my faith in God. What did I believe? Why did I go to church? Our friends, Nancy and Bill, had peace in their lives. They talked about God as if they knew Him. Why not me? To me, they were an example of God's love. I liked being with them. There was a peace in their lives that I wanted, but did not have. They had their problems, but I knew they trusted in the Lord.

Every week, Nancy would call and ask, "How are you doing, At?" I knew she prayed for us.

"Why," I questioned, "don't I have that kind of peace with the Lord? What is wrong with me? I go to church, I have accepted Jesus into my heart, yet, I have no peace," I continued. "I cannot really say that I trust God! I need to know," I thought. "I really want that."

I began to pray out loud, "God, if You are there, I want to know You. Either You are real and You can help us, or You are not, and then I don't want to go to church anymore. So God, if You are there, I want to know You!"

At that very instant, something happened to me. God quickened my spirit, and hope and inner joy flowed in. Suddenly, the voice on the radio, which I had previously been oblivious to, called out these words, "If anyone needs prayer, go to God. He will hear you."

"Prayer! Of course! I can pray to God, and He will hear me," I realized. Amazingly, I had listened to that particular radio station before but never heard a minister on it.

It was like I received a present. I don't know how, but suddenly the trees in our yard looked greener; the sky looked bluer. Something amazing took place in my spirit, and hope flooded in. I could not wait until my husband came home for lunch. I wanted to share with him the wonderful experience I had with the Lord that morning.

I called Simen at his job, wondering what I should tell him. All I could say was, "When you come home, Simen, I will share some good news with you."

"Tell me now," he said. "Why can't you tell me?"

"No," I said, "I'll wait until you come home. It is too important to tell you over the telephone." With that I hung up, wondering what I would say to him. We never talked about the Lord, so I did not know how he would react.

When I saw Simen coming home that day, I ran to open the door. "Well," he said, "what's the good news?"

"Simen," I started, "we can go to the Lord in prayer and He will help us!" With that, I looked at him to see how he was going to react. He looked back at me intently and said, "I know." Two simple words were all it took. God started to work in his heart. No big theological discussion, no argument about it, but simply, "I know He will help us."

That was all it took for God to begin to work in him. My husband was so open to the Lord that day. He listened intently while I shared with him what had happened that morning. He believed what I told him. This was God! Later, he said, "You know, At, as you shared with me what took place that morning, how the Lord had put hope in your heart, the same thing happened to me." God met my husband and did a work in his heart.

It was the beginning of a whole new life for both of us and for our family. Our problems were not solved that day, but we knew to go with them to the Lord. There was hope and an expectation.

That evening a friend called and asked, "Attie, do you want to go with me to a Bible study tonight?"

"What is the topic?" I asked her.

"Prayer," she said. "Prayer, and it is going to be good. A lady from New Zealand is there to minister. You want to go, At?"

"Yes," I said. The subjects were Prayer Changes Things and How to Hear the Voice of God. Both of them were just what I needed to hear. I wanted God to speak to me!

That evening the lady from New Zealand shared that praying to the Lord is like picking up the phone and saying, "Hi, God, I need to talk to You. I need Your help!" She said she prays about everything, even if she is in her car and gets lost, she asks the Lord where to go. And the Lord always helps her. Nothing is too big or too small for the Lord.

I listened to her and thought, "If the Lord speaks to her, He will speak to me." Right there in that class I prayed, asking the Lord to help me to hear His voice.

That evening I learned that God still speaks to His people. He spoke to Adam and Eve in the Garden of Eden. He spoke to Abraham, who is called a friend of God. He spoke to Noah, who built a boat, and He wants to speak to you and me, too!

The Lord will bring hope to you, too. Perhaps, like me back then, you have nowhere to go. Maybe you do not know the Lord, but you want to. As you read this, stop for a minute and ask God to help you, to reveal Himself to you as He did to me. All you have to say is:

> *Dear God,*
>
> *I want to know You. I believe that You died for my sins on the cross.*
> *Come into my heart. I give You my life.*
> *In Jesus' name, amen.*

And Jesus said to Him, "If you can!" All things are possible to him who believes.

—Mark 9:23, TLB

4

I BELIEVE IN MIRACLES

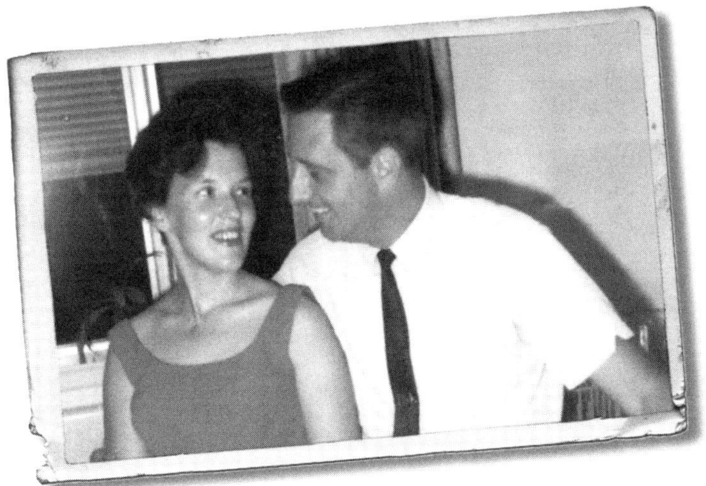

Attie and Simen at the Terhune kitchen

Therefore if any man be in Christ, he is a new creature: old things are passed away; behold, all things are become new.
—2 Corinthians 5:17, KJV

A WHOLE NEW WORLD opened up for Simen and me. Perceiving in our spirits that there was more, we asked, "Where do we go from here?" Everything was so new to us. There was an awareness of God's presence, a knowing that He heard our prayers. It was exciting! We never before discussed God's Word or even prayed together. But now it was altogether different at our home. We learned to share our faith in God. We prayed and read the Bible together. And there was an expectancy that there was more. God has actually given us His Spirit to tell us about the wonderful free gift of grace and blessing that God has given us and is about to give us as we look to Him for everything.

> No mere man has ever seen, heard, or even imagined what wonderful things God has ready for those who love the Lord. But we know about these things because God has sent his Spirit to tell us, and his Spirit searches out and shows us all of God's deepest secrets. No one can really know what anyone else is thinking or what he is really like except that person himself. And no one can know God's thoughts except God's own Spirit.
>
> —1 Corinthians 2:9–11, TLB

We can see this demonstrated as Jesus appeared to His disciples on the road to Emmaus after the Resurrection. The stone was rolled away and Jesus was not in the tomb. Luke 24:14 says, "And [the disciples] talked together of all these things which had happened." While they conversed, Jesus drew near and walked with them, but they did not recognize Him. "And He said to them, 'What kind of conversation is this that you have with one another as you walk and are sad?'" (Luke 24:17). So they told Jesus everything that had taken place, including how Jesus was condemned to death and crucified. They explained that they had hoped that Jesus was going to redeem Israel. Then Jesus began to speak to them concerning all that had to take place, "And beginning at Moses and all the Prophets, He expounded to them in all the Scriptures the things concerning Himself.…Then their eyes were opened and they knew Him" (Luke 24:27, 31). The passage "they knew him" describes a revelation by the Holy Spirit.

That day our spirits were opened, and it was like a revelation had taken place in our hearts. We were expecting to hear from God. My husband and I sat around the table talking and sharing about the Lord when a particular incident that had taken place five years earlier came into my memory.

It was dinnertime and I had forgotten the nutmeg for the cauliflower I was preparing that day. (You have to live at our home to know how important the nutmeg is. The cauliflower just does not taste the same if you do not season it with nutmeg.) As I ran out of the house, I called out to my husband saying, "I'll be right back, Simen! Watch the food for me on the stove so it won't burn!"

As I walked into the grocery store, our neighbor approached me and said, "Hi, Attie. Did you know Oral Roberts is in town tomorrow? Why don't you go hear him?"

I looked at her, not knowing how to respond. Frankly, I was embarrassed, thinking, "Oral Roberts? Why should I go there?" I knew who he was; he prayed for the sick. Thinking back, I had seen him on television, and since I did not believe that healings were for today, I usually turned off the TV when he came on.

As if she knew what I was thinking, she said, "Attie, God still heals today! He healed my daughter, Becky. She was born with a birth defect in her back fifteen years ago."

My thoughts raced ahead of me. I knew Becky very well. She was our babysitter some years prior, and I knew there was nothing wrong with her back.

"When Becky was two years old," her mother continued, "I went with her to see Oral Roberts. He prayed for her, and God completely healed her." Listening, I could not really say I disbelieved her, but it did not touch me, either. All I could think was, "I have to get home or the food will burn." After politely saying good-bye, I went my way.

Now, five years later, as I was relating this incident to Simen, he said, "Why don't you give her a call?"

"Me? Call her? After five years?" I was indifferent to our neighbor when she talked to me in that store five years ago. And in the meantime, we had moved away and lost all contact with each other. But despite some misgivings, I phoned her anyway.

After exchanging a short greeting, I asked her to repeat what she had told me five years earlier, about the Lord healing her little girl. There was a momentary silence on the other end of the line. Then I heard laughing. "What has happened to you, Attie?" she asked, and I shared with her what the Lord had done for Simen and me.

"Praise the Lord!" was her reply. Then she began to tell me again how the Lord still heals today.

Did we dare ask the questions, Does God still heal incurable diseases? Would He for our son? Now, five years later, I was willing to listen to the Lord. Life had become different for us, with God regulating our day-to-day existence. We experienced God's presence in a fuller measure. There was still sadness when Simon was in pain, but with God there was a difference.

A few days later I was in the kitchen making coffee and my husband walked in. Pointing to a book in his hands, he said, "Attie, where did you get this book?"

"Oh," I said, not very enthusiastically, "Mom gave it to me." Two months earlier my mother had given me a book entitled *I Believe in Miracles* by Kathryn Kuhlman, saying, "Why don't you read this book, At?" I had picked up the book once and, after reading a couple of lines, closed it, thinking, "Oh, it is about miracles. I don't want to read it." Not understanding the wonderful, miraculous power of God, I forgot about it until that evening.

"Why would he want to read a book like that?" I wondered. But God was not through with us, yet. My husband took the book in the living room and began to read, not at the beginning, but somewhere near the middle. He did not check to see who the author was. The story he read was about a boy who was miraculously healed by God of perthes disease. The boy was nine years old at the time of the healing.

After reading the story, Simen closed the book and turned on the television at 10:30 p.m. To his surprise, a program called *I Believe in Miracles* was on—the same title as the book he just was reading! The host on the program was Miss Kathryn Kuhlman. My husband took a closer look at the book he had been reading a few minutes earlier and began to get excited when he noticed that the author of the book and the lady on the program were one and the same. That was a startling coincidence!

"Attie," he called, "You have to come here." After he explained to me what had just taken place, both of us watched the program intently, not knowing what would happen next. To our surprise, Miss Kuhlman's guest was none other than the boy my husband had just been reading about! He was now twenty-nine years old and still healed, twenty years later.

As the program continued, we noticed that there was a striking similarity between Simon and the man who was healed as a nine-year-old boy. Both diseases had started with complaints about pain in their left legs. We were amazed, and our hearts were open to the Lord.

"Can this be true, God?" we asked.

At the end of the program, the announcer gave the time and the location of the next healing service: July 17, 1969. After that my husband said, "That is where we are going!" We had never heard of Kathryn Kuhlman. We did not even know she had a program on television every Sunday called *I Believe in Miracles*, but God knew, and He arranged all the circumstances that evening.

After seeing the program on television, I became more interested in the book my mother had given me.

"Simen," I said, "can I read it?" And as I began, I could not put it down. It was fantastic. A whole new world opened up for me when I read one story after another of how the Lord had healed people of all kinds of diseases. Seeds of faith were sown in our hearts as both of us read the book. After we finished, we wanted to know how the Lord still healed today. We bought book after book, and together with studying the Word of God, we learned and grew more in the Word. We became closer to God and each other, and our spiritual eyes were more and more open to the fact that God was interested in all our everyday affairs. Oh, what a discovery! We could not learn enough about Jesus, who healed the sick and came to set free those who were in need.

We also discovered a Christian bookstore nearby. Every week you could find us in that store, buying books on all kinds of subjects relating to the kingdom of God. We were so hungry for more of God. We introduced our children to Christian books and music. They enjoyed going with us to the bookstore, always coming home with something new to read or listen to. We all had a great time exploring what was so new to all of us. Christian books and music and, of course, coloring books for the little ones.

Before we knew it, Sunday came along, the day of the miracle service. We did not know what to expect. The whole family went, full of expectation and excitement. Could this be the day that Simon would be healed? Simon had told his doctor, days earlier, "God is going to heal me. I am going to a healing service!" With that he looked at the doctor's face. The doctor looked at him and did not respond, for which I was thankful, because I knew he was not a believer in miracles. Yet, listening to our son that day, I began to worry. What if Simon did not get healed? What would it do to his faith? Many doubts and questions enveloped me. I did not want to sow doubt into Simon's mind, but rather to encourage him that with the Lord all things are possible. And with that I left it in God's hands.

Also, I could not help but think what our friends Bill and Nancy had shared with us the evening before. It was a week earlier when they came over to our car on the way out of church. We were about to leave when I heard someone call our names, "At and Simen, how are you all doing?"

Turning around, we saw Bill and Nancy approach us. All excited, I said, "You'll never guess what happened to us!" We shared everything that had happened in the last few weeks, including the book, *I Believe in Miracles*, and the television program of the same name. I told them that we were going to the miracle service the following Sunday. They looked at us in amazement. "You believe that Simon is going to get healed Sunday?" Bill asked.

"Yes," I replied. "Why not?"

Bill and Nancy looked at each other. "Can we come over Saturday evening before you go and pray with you?"

"Sure," we said. "We will see you Saturday."

As we left for our home we wondered why they acted so strange. That was not at all the Bill and Nancy I knew. In the past they had always encouraged us to look to the Lord for everything. Now they acted so weary.

When they came over that Saturday, they truly rejoiced with us as we shared our commitment to God. But then they became cautious, saying, "Yes, we believe God can heal Simon, but we must not forget to leave it in the hands of God."

> Not my will, but yours be done.
>
> —Luke 22:42, NIV

Wow, I could not get away from that verse for the next six months.

Driving down to the miracle service that day, all those thoughts ran through my mind. Tears began streaming down my face as I finally realized it was the Lord I had resisted all those years. My husband looked at me, touching my hand. That day I asked the Lord to forgive me of my sins of not listening to Him sooner. Over and over again the Lord had sent people to me to tell me that Jesus is "the same yesterday and today and forever" (Heb. 13:8, NIV), and that "all things are possible" to those that believe (Matt. 19:26, NIV). I thought about one

Bible passage in particular, where Jesus said, "The Spirit of the Lord God is upon me, because the Lord has anointed me to bring good news to the suffering and afflicted. He has sent me to comfort the brokenhearted, to announce liberty to captives, and to open the eyes of the blind" (Isa. 61:1, TLB). I had not believed. All of this went through my mind as we were driving to the miracle service. Was this the way back to God? Now as I needed Him, I learned He is a patient and merciful God.

When we arrived at the miracle service at ten o'clock, thousands of people were already standing in line waiting to get in. We had never seen anything like this before. People came in wheelchairs and on crutches, needing healing. We had never gone to church like this. We saw many people praying and worshiping God, all before the service had even begun.

As we looked around, a lady walked up and introduced herself to us, "Hi, my name is Ruth. Who are you?" After we introduced ourselves, she asked us why we were there. We began to share with her that we came for a healing for our son Simon.

"What is wrong with him?" she asked. "Because I believe that the Lord is going to do something for you people!"

"Simon is diagnosed with scleroderma," I said to her, "and we came for a healing."

"There is a lady who works with us," Ruth said. "She works around the corner at the wheelchair section. God has healed her of scleroderma, and now she works at the special section for the handicapped and the disabled people." She looked at us and said, "Why don't you go there? Tell her I sent you, and from now on you do not have to stand in line; you can go right in. And remember, God is going to do something special for you people!"

After we introduced ourselves to Mrs. Bennet, she shared her testimony with us of how the Lord had healed her of scleroderma many years ago. We were so encouraged, and the service had not even started yet. After we found seats on the top balcony, we were expecting something from God.

As the service began, seven thousand people began to worship the Lord. The choir began to sing "He Touched Me":

> He touched me, He touched me,
> and oh the joy that floods my soul.
> Something happened and now I know
> He touched me and made me whole. [2]

To me it sounded like a chorus straight from heaven. We had never experienced a church service like that before. What impressed me was the attitude of worship and praise, and the moments of absolute silence in the audience of such a vast number of people.

I looked around and it was like a scene right out of heaven. In heaven we are going to praise the Lord. The apostle John recorded a scene out of heaven when God told him to write down what he had been permitted to see:

> Then a voice came from the throne, saying, "Praise our God, all you His servants and those who fear Him, both small and great!" And I heard as it were, the voice of a great multitude, as the sound of many waters and as the sound of mighty thunderings, saying, "Alleluia!" For the Lord God Omnipotent reigns!...."And [John said] I fell at His feet to worship Him."
>
> —Revelation 19:5–6, 10, NASB

You can only worship Him when you are in the presence of God. There are no words, just total surrender in worship and praise. As seven thousand people worshiped the Lord, healings

2. HE TOUCHED ME/Williams J. Gaither/Gaither Music Company (ASCAP)/All rights controlled by Gaither Copyright Management. Used by permission.

took place all around us, right where the people were sitting. Miss Kuhlman never gave a sermon that day. She started to give a sermon, but had to stop because people were being healed all around us.

Behind us was a man who traded seats with me so we could all sit together. All of a sudden, his deaf ears opened up. God had healed him! We knew he was deaf because when we had arrived that morning, Simen had tried to communicate with him on paper because he could not speak. When the Lord opened his ears, it scared him, and he began to scream and put his fingers in his ears. He was totally healed that day. God healed him!

When I was confronted with healings all around me, I had to ask myself, "Do I believe God still heals today?" This was the day that I was truly faced with the reality of the living God. It was like someone put a floodlight in my heart, and I did not like what I saw. "Oh, God," I said, "help my unbelief! I want to believe. I want to know. Please, God, help me!" I prayed.

I had heard Bible stories all my life, gone to a Christian school and Sunday school, and yet when confronted with miracles, I did not believe. The Lord had to give me the faith to believe.

For the first time in my life I realized I was hiding behind the false phrase "healing was only for the apostolic age." It was not a pretty picture. And I brought it all to the Lord in prayer, and I asked God to help me. Only then can we be sure that, "If any man will do his will, he shall know of the doctrine, whether it be of God, or whether I speak of myself" (John 7:17, KJV). The emphasis here is on the phrase "will do His will." Then faith can grow a living dependence on God's kind of faith. It is the Lord who brings faith to maturity in us.

> And I am sure that God who began the good work within you will keep right on helping you grow in his grace until his task within you is finally finished on that day when Jesus Christ returns.
>
> —Philippians 1:6, TLB

> For God is at work within you, helping you want to obey him, and then helping you do what he wants.
>
> —Philippians 2:13, TLB

When we arrived home that day, Simon was not healed, but many changes were to take place in us. First, I began to realize there was more to being a Christian than I had thought. A hunger for more of the Lord began to grip me. At home, a greater awareness of God became evident. At the dinner table, when it was time for my husband or me to read the Scriptures, one of us would say, "Now it is my turn." Then the other would say, "No, it is my turn," and we all would laugh! Later we realized how much our children had picked up from our sharing God's Word with one another. It was the beginning of a whole new way of life for all of us.

There were many delightful moments despite Simon's illness, moments that brought us closer together as a family. Every evening Simon had to do physical exercises. We all made up games to play—Jackie, Simon, Michael, Yvonne, and me. They could not wait for me to spread out a blanket on the floor and see who could do ten push-ups. Or who was the first to crawl across the living room floor. It was a close, recreational time for all of us, with their dad as the referee and me always the loser, to the great pleasure of the rest of the family.

I began to look at our children more closely and used every opportunity to teach them about the Lord. What could have been a trying and difficult time for all of us was turned into ways of instilling God's truth into our children's lives. We saw what was really important—that we were not just living for now, but for eternity. It was as if we had stopped our everyday, busy lives to take an account of where we were going. It brought not only my husband and me closer to God, but also our children.

Exactly how close was brought home to me when Simon returned from a Christmas party at school when he was six years old. Walking over to the Christmas tree in front of our window, he took a neatly wrapped piece of chocolate out of his pocket. I watched him put the chocolate on the tree, thinking nothing of it, until some time later when the phone rang. It was Simon calling from a friend's house. "Mom," he asked, "can you go to the Christmas tree and see if Jesus already took out His chocolate? It's for His birthday!" I could not help but smile to know that Jesus was that real to him.

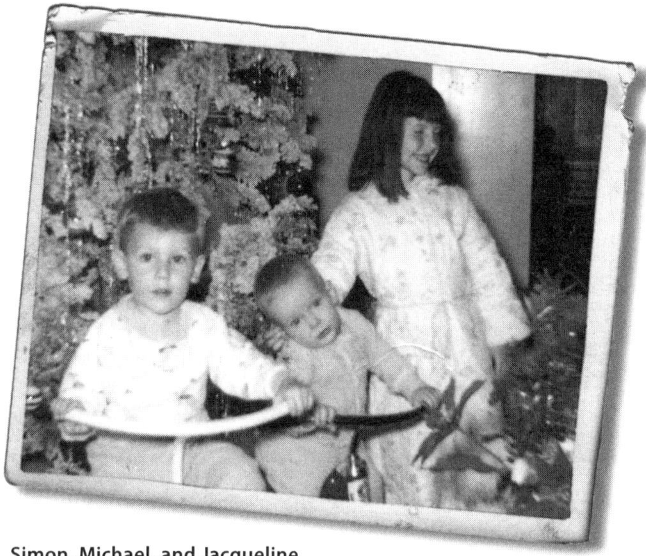

Simon, Michael, and Jacqueline

What happiness for those whose guilt has been forgiven! What joys when sins are covered over! What relief for those who have confessed their sins and God has cleared their record.

—Psalm 32:1–2, TLB

5

PEACE WITH GOD

IT WAS THE opening of the charismatic clinic at Melodyland Christian Center. The entire family went, hoping this would be the evening that God would heal Simon. Our hopes were high. All of us arrived early so we could sit together, but as usual, many people were already there before the service started.

The doors opened at six o'clock and the people literally streamed in. Sitting in that church for the first time, we felt the overwhelming presence of God. "God is in this place, too," I thought, "just as He was at the miracle service and the Monday evening prayer service at North Hollywood Assembly of God."

Kathryn Kuhlman was going to minister that night, and my prayer was, "Please, God, heal Simon." The choir began to worship and the audience joined in joyfully. I quickly got caught up in worshiping the Lord. When Miss Kuhlman began to preach, my thoughts went to Simon. Looking at him next to me, I pleaded once again, "Please, God, heal Simon!" When the altar call was given, my husband said to me, "At, are you going with me for prayer?"

"Sure," I said, thinking he wanted prayer for Simon for a healing. So we all went to the front for prayer. After the minister had taken us to the prayer room, my husband asked, "What must I do to be saved?"

I was startled! "My husband? Not saved?" I thought. Why, he had gone to church most of his life! He was water baptized at the age of fifteen, and yet he did not know Jesus as his personal Savior? I could not believe my ears.

I had been so absorbed in prayer for Simon our son that I had not understood until then that my husband might not be saved. "But, he went to church," I reasoned. "He was an elder in our church, he and I talked about the Lord, and he was hungry for more of the Lord!" I thought. Could it be that he was not saved?

I listened as the counselor began to answer my husband's questions. The counselor was a chemist by trade, and so was my husband. They both were precise and detailed in their explanations. The counselor knew the Word well, I noticed.

> For what will a man be profited if he gains the whole world, and loses his own soul?
>
> —Mark 8:36

I listened, still amazed that I had not known my husband was not saved! But God knew! The minister continued, "If God granted us everything we asked for, it would be disastrous. We do not always know what is best for us, for we are too time conscious. But God looks at the total picture of our lives, '"For My thoughts are not your thoughts, nor are your ways My ways," says the Lord'" (Isa. 55:8).

As I listened to the counselor with somewhat mixed emotions, I heard my husband ask, "How can I know that I am saved? And what happens when I sin again tomorrow?" He had a terrible time with the concept of sin, for he could not understand how the Lord could forgive his sins once and for all.

The counselor told him not to worry about it at that time, and that he would go with him through the Bible and ask the Lord to make it real to him. "Your old nature," he said, "cannot serve God, 'but the natural man does not receive the things of the Spirit of God, for they are foolishness to him; nor can he know them, because they are spiritually discerned.'[3] That is why Jesus said, 'You must be born again.'[4] The infinitive *be* is passive; it shows that it is something that must be done for us. No one can *birth* himself. It is a gift from God. Nicodemus could not understand it. He asked twice, but could not understand how a man can be born again. And Jesus answered him, 'Man can only reproduce human life, but the Holy Spirit gives new life from heaven.'[5] Being born again is the work of the Holy Spirit. It is God's part. Our part is to receive Him: 'But as many as received Him, to them He gave the power to become the sons of God.'"[6]

"But how can I know?" my husband asked.

"Well," the counselor said, "we all have sinned and come short of the glory of God.[7] No one is without sin. The Bible says, 'God, who commanded the light to shine out of darkness, hath shined in our hearts, to give the light of the knowledge of the glory of God in the face of Jesus Christ.'[8] It also says that 'the eyes of your understanding being enlightened,'[9] you change. You understand the things before you thought were foolish, for now you live by faith. Your whole mental process is changed," the counselor continued. "God becomes the center of your being. Also, your heart undergoes a radical change. Ezekiel 36:26 says, 'I will give you a new heart and put a new spirit within you; I will take the heart of stone out of your flesh and give you a heart of flesh,'" the counselor said. "You receive a new heart; a heart that loves God. Your new nature loves God and the things pertaining to God."

The counselor explained to Simen, "The moment that you are born again, you receive a divine impartation of a new nature,

3. Corinthians 2:14
4. John 3:7
5. John 3:6, TLB
6. John 1:12, KJV
7. See Romans 3:23
8. 2 Corinthians 4:6, KJV
9. Ephesians 1:18, KJV

and you are justified in God's sight. *Justified* means 'just as if I'd never sinned.' The Lord does this. It is an act of God. And all of your sins will be forgiven—the ones you did yesterday, today, and tomorrow," he stated.

"Really?" my husband asked. "God will forgive all my sins? Again and again?"

"Yes," the counselor answered. "And, 1 John 1:9 says, 'If we confess our sins to him, he can be depended on to forgive us and to cleanse us from every wrong.'[10] See, it is like this. Paul says, 'I passed on to you right from the first what had been told to me, that Christ died for our sins just as the Scriptures said he would, and that he was buried, and three days afterwards He arose from the grave just as the prophets foretold.'[11] It is for whosoever will. No one is excluded!" the counselor continued.

At this point I interrupted the conversation. "Simen, we've got to get home. It is late!" My husband looked at me and said, "Not yet, Attie. Just wait a minute, will you?" His commitment was total, and the counselor went on as if nothing had happened. "Now we can come to the Father, and if we confess and believe that Jesus died on the cross for our sins and rose again the third day, He will forgive us of our sins." The counselor continued explaining to Simen, "Not *maybe*; He will, just as you are with all your faults—and that is the good news! You cannot earn it or say, 'I first have to clean up my life.' No, you come as you are, and you give your life to God and ask Him to help you. The thief on the cross had faith when he said, 'This man, Jesus, does not deserve to die. He has done nothing wrong. We are receiving what we deserve for our deeds. 'Jesus,' he said, 'remember me when You come in your Kingdom!' And Jesus said to him, 'Today you shall be with Me in Paradise.'[12] All this man had to offer was faith!" the counselor continued.

---

10. TLB
11. 1 Corinthians 15:3-4, TLB
12. See Luke 23:42-43

I listened in utter amazement. It was good that God oversaw the entire situation and not me. He knew what we needed. I had not the slightest idea until both my husband and the counselor began to pray, "Dear heavenly Father, forgive my sins. I am sorry for my sins. I ask You to cleanse me. I receive You now as my personal Savior. In Jesus' name, amen."

When we walked out of church that night, I asked my husband, "What happened to you tonight?" He looked at me joyfully and said, "I am saved!" and with that he made a jump and laughed!

Then I knew that something had happened to him. He was so joyful and so happy. Later he told me that when I asked him that evening what had taken place, something took place in his spirit and he knew that he knew that he was born again. He was a new person in Christ.

All those years I did not know my husband was not saved. But God knew. My eyes were opened to the startling realization that you can sit in church, be a member of a church, even work in church, and not know the Lord. You can be a religious person and not have a personal relationship with God. This happened to Nicodemus, a religious man who knew the Scriptures, but did not know Jesus, so Jesus explained to him: "What I am telling you so earnestly is this: unless one is born of water and the Spirit, he cannot enter the kingdom of God. Men can only produce human life, but the Holy Spirit gives new life from heaven, so don't be surprised at my statement that you must be born again."[13]

This was an eye-opener for me as a mom. I realized then that also our children needed to be born again. Children have a tremendous capacity for knowing the Lord. It is so easy to lead a little child to the Lord. I had the privilege to lead all of our four children to the Lord.

---

13. See John 3:5, 7, TLB

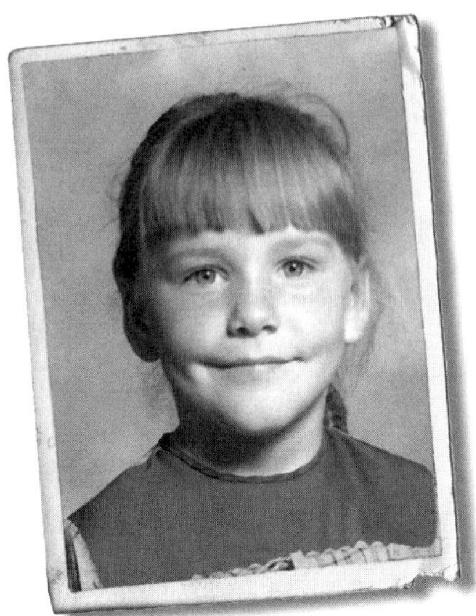

Yvonne

Yvonne, who was six years old at the time, came to me one day and said, "Mom, I want to be water baptized. May I?"

"Are you sure, Yvonne?" I asked.

"Yes, Mom, I want to."

On the following Sunday evening, Yvonne was baptized. I went with her and held her on my lap, waiting for her turn to be baptized. She was singing to the Lord. It was so special, and when it was her turn to be baptized, the minister asked her, "Well, Yvonne, how long have you known the Lord?"

With a big smile she said, "All my life." We thanked the Lord for this. I felt such thankfulness to the Lord for opening up our spiritual eyes. Looking at our daughter, such a beautiful girl, and hearing her say, "I've known the Lord all my life," was a blessing!

In God's Word, it says that Jesus called a child to Himself and stood him in their midst, and said, "Truly I say to you, unless you are converted and become like children, you shall not enter the kingdom of heaven.... And whoever receives one such child in

My name receives Me" (Matt. 18:3, 5, NAS). Children are such an example of what we should be like: open and trusting, believing the Lord. God gives us many opportunities to talk to and teach our children about the Lord, to pray with them, and see God answering their prayers.

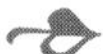

At 5:59 a.m. on Tuesday, February 9, 1971, an earthquake hit California, and anyone who lived in California that particular day will never forget it. We were asleep when the beds rattled. We were holding on for dear life. Our front door blew open, and it was like a fireball went right through our house. My in-laws were visiting us from Holland, and my father-in-law said, "I am going home! That's it!"

After we all calmed down, we went to the living room, turned on the TV, and heard the news that we were struck by an earthquake of a magnitude of 6.5 on the Richter scale. Experts at Caltech Seismology Laboratory said the quake centered about ten miles east of Newhall, California. It was a wake-up call, literally and figuratively, for many people.

We personally knew quite a few people who made a decision for the Lord that day, as did our oldest daughter, Jacqueline. She went to a Bible study at our church that evening, as she did every Thursday. But this was special. The young people in her study wanted to share and pray about the earthquake that had struck that day. When Jacqueline came home that evening, she had many questions about God and about eternity.

"What happens after we die?" she asked me. "And Mom," she continued, "I don't know that I am saved or where I am going." Big tears streamed down her face. I looked at my daughter and asked, "What makes you think that?"

"Well," she replied, "you know that you are saved! Dad knows! Simon knows. Everyone knows, but me. I don't know!" That evening I had the privilege, as a mom, to lead our oldest daughter to the Lord. There is no greater joy than to pray with your children to receive Christ. After we prayed together, she broke out in a smile. She dried her tears and said, "I am saved. I just invited Jesus into my heart!"

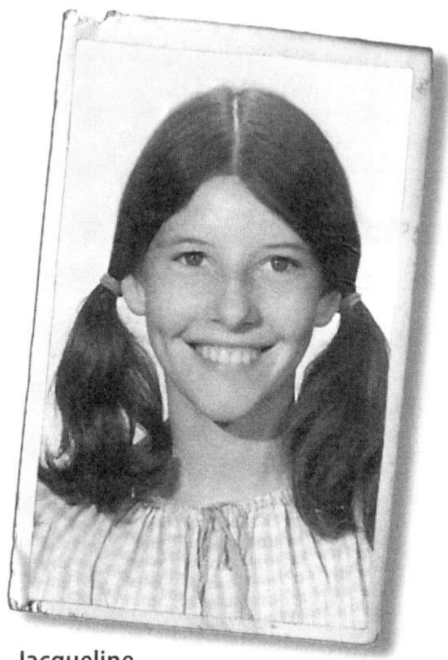

Jacqueline

Now the Lord is the Spirit; and where the Spirit of the Lord is, there is liberty.

—2 Corinthians 3:17, NASB

6

THERE IS LIBERTY

THERE WAS A small Pentecostal church in the little town where I grew up. People warned me not to go to that church because, they said, wild things happened there. Some claimed that after people were healed in that church, they climbed the poles. (Why they climbed them I never knew, but I wanted no part of it, so I never went in.) Ironically, years later when I needed to be closer to the Lord, guess where He led me? Yes, to a Pentecostal church.

When we arrived for our first visit, we really felt at home. People all around us were worshiping and praising the Lord, and we deeply felt the presence of God. After the singing stopped, the pastor encouraged people to give their personal testimony, and one by one they stood up and thanked the Lord for what He had done in their lives. What really impressed me was the freedom of the people in praising the Lord. There was such a joy and liberty. It reminded me of the Scripture that says, "And where the Spirit of the Lord is, there is liberty" (2 Cor. 3:17). The Lord had answered their prayers for the salvation of loved ones. An alcoholic husband had been set free. He had been addicted for thirteen years, and the Lord instantly delivered him. Incurable diseases were healed. It was like seeing the gospel in action.

Faith began to rise in me and I thought, "If God does that for them, He can do it for me." I had seen the power of God in the Kathryn Kuhlman service, but I did not realize until that evening that the Lord worked in other churches as well.

As I was sitting there, I remember thinking, "Why was I so afraid to go to a Pentecostal church? I have not seen any emotional outbreaks or people climbing poles, as I had been warned. No wonder the devil did not want me here. He knew the power of God was in this place, and these people serve a living God." I felt one with them; they loved and served the same God I did.

As we came to the end of the service, something happened that startled me. The minister began leading people in worship, and while they were praising the Lord, he encouraged them to worship God in their prayer language. I was absolutely amazed. I had never heard of speaking in tongues or the baptism with the Holy Spirit. Yet, I was familiar with it, because I did the same thing when I was a child when I accepted Jesus as my Savior. Then, some time later, I felt the overwhelming presence of God around me, and I felt compelled to speak in another language, not understanding that it was one of the manifestations of the Holy Spirit.

There were times when I wondered why I could speak so fluently in another language, thinking I was the only one in this world who could do this. Until that evening, I had never told anyone of that experience.

When we came home that night, my husband asked me how I liked the service.

"Beautiful," I said, looking for words to tell him of my experience. "Simen," I said, "I have to tell you something. Those people tonight in church, praying in tongues, did the same thing I did when I was a child." Then I explained what had taken place years earlier.

My husband looked at me and began to laugh. "Oh," he said, "you have been baptized with the Holy Spirit! Let me hear you speak in tongues!"

"No way," I exclaimed. I felt afraid and did not think speaking in tongues was funny. What would I say? To me it was simply a play language. The last time I could remember using it was when our oldest daughter, Jackie, was four years old. I remember asking her, "Jackie, do you want to hear your mom speak in another language?" And Jackie, eyes opened, looked up at me expectantly. All this came to my memory when Simen and I were talking.

"Oh, Simen," I explained excitedly, "I was close to the Lord then. Remember the children's Bible stories I bought?"

"Yes," he said, "I remember."

Those books had cost a lot of money. A man had come to our door and asked if he could come in and show me some children's Bible books.

"Sure," I said, and invited him in. He came in with a complete set of Bible stories for children, covering Genesis to Revelation. Looking through them, I knew I loved them. He also showed me a set of books with character-building stories for small children. I loved them immediately, too.

"How much do the books cost?" I asked.

"All together, $135," he said.

"I will buy them," I said, convinced that this was what I wanted to read to my children.

"Don't you have to talk it over with your husband first?" he asked.

"No," I said. "It will be all right with him."

"I will leave you one book and the rest will be sent to you in about six weeks," he told me.

After he left, I began reading to our daughter Jackie, and we both loved the stories. Later on, I read them to all our children. It was in moments like those that I felt close to the Lord, and it was also the time I spoke in tongues.

"Well," my husband said, "then you were baptized in the Holy Spirit as a child."

"You really believe that?" I asked.

"Yes, I do," my husband said.

We had many questions, and we searched the Scriptures, asking the Lord to teach us. We also read books, such as *The*

Holy Spirit and You by Dennis and Rita Bennett and *Overflowing Life* by Robert C. Frost, which were of a great help and encouragement to both of us. Simen and I had a lot of catching up to do, and so many things to learn. We stayed up late in the evening discussing what we had just read about. I did not want to pray in tongues until I understood its meaning and purpose. It is amazing to me now to think back and be able to see the hand of God on my life and to realize that the Lord was in this place and that place, while I took everything for granted. I can see now that even though I was not faithful, God was. I truly can say, Thank you, God!

In searching the Scriptures, I became convinced how important the Holy Spirit's work is. Before Jesus ascended to heaven, He gave His apostles some important words of instruction:

> Wait for the Promise of the Father…for John truly baptized with water, but you shall be baptized with the Holy Spirit not many days from now.
>
> —Acts 1:4–5

Ten days after the ascension of Jesus, 120 believers were together worshiping and praising God. On the day of Pentecost (a religious feast of the Jews), the Holy Spirit was poured out, and a rushing wind filled the whole house where they were sitting.

> And they were all filled with the Holy Spirit and began to speak with other tongues, as the Spirit gave them utterance.
>
> —Acts 2:4

The term *other tongues* here refers to spoken languages, unknown to the speakers but known by others. Many of the people who were listening that day were devout Jews from all over the world, coming together for the religious celebrations.

The out-of-towners were amazed to hear their own language being spoken by the disciples.

> Tongues are for a sign, not to those who believe but to unbelievers.
>
> —1 Corinthians 14:22

> Others mocking said, "They are full of new wine." But Peter, standing up with the eleven, raised his voice and said to them, "Men of Judea and all who dwell in Jerusalem, let this be known to you, and heed my words. For these are not drunk, as you suppose, since it is only the third hour of the day. But this is what was spoken by the prophet Joel: 'And it shall come to pass in the last days, says God, That I will pour out My Spirit on all flesh.'"
>
> —Acts 2:13–17

After Peter had preached the Word, three thousand people received Jesus as their Savior and were baptized that same day.

As I began to study the Word, I began to understand that there are two kinds of tongues, the first being for private devotions, mentioned in 1 Corinthians 14:2: "For one who speaks in a tongue speaks not to men but to God" (RSV). The apostle Paul says, "For if I pray in a tongue, my spirit prays" (1 Cor. 14:14, RSV). In Acts 2:4, for instance, the "other tongues" are languages used in lands other than Palestine, and were only understood by the people who spoke that language.

In 1 Corinthians 12:6–11, where the subject is the gifts of the Spirit, it is talking about the gift of healing, wisdom, and miracles, among others. They are gifts given as the Spirit wills at the moment. Verse 30 says, "Do all have the gift of healing? Do all speak in tongues? Do all interpret?" (1 Cor. 12:30, NIV). When someone receives the gift of tongues in a church meeting, one also has to interpret that message. But the apostle Paul goes on to say, "I thank my God I speak with tongues more than you all" (1 Cor. 14:18).

In Acts 8:14–17 we read, "When the apostles back in Jerusalem heard that the people of Samaria had accepted God's message, they sent down Peter and John. As soon as they arrived, they began praying for these new Christians to receive the Holy Spirit, for as yet he had not come upon any of them. For they had only been baptized in the name of the Lord Jesus. Then Peter and John laid their hands upon these believers, and they received the Holy Spirit" (TLB). No mention of tongues is made here, but Simon the sorcerer saw that the Spirit was bestowed through the laying on of the apostle's hands, and he offered them money for the gift. (See Acts 8:18.)

The next episode is on the Damascus road where Saul met Jesus, who said to him, "Saul, Saul, why are you persecuting Me?" (Acts 9:4). After his encounter with Jesus, Saul was blinded, unable to see for three days. Then the Lord sent to him a disciple named Ananias who laid hands on Saul and said, "Brother Paul, the Lord Jesus, who appeared to you on the road, has sent me so that you may be filled with the Holy Spirit and get your sight back" (Acts 9:17, TLB).

Some eleven years after Pentecost, the Holy Spirit was also given to the Gentiles in a town called Caesarea Philippi, the center of the Roman occupation forces. In that town lived a Roman officer named Cornelius who believed in God. One afternoon as he was praying, he had a vision and was told by an angel of the Lord to send for Peter, who would instruct him what to do. (See Acts 10:6.) So Cornelius called for his servants and godly soldiers and sent them to Joppa, where Peter was staying.

In the meantime, Peter was praying, and God spoke to him through a series of visions and direct instructions to go with the Roman soldiers to Cornelius's house. In those days, Peter, a Jew, never would have gone to a Gentile's home without the instruction of God, even to tell them about Jesus. When a

Gentile wanted to receive Christ, he first had to become a Jew and go through the requirements of the Jewish law. When Peter arrived at Cornelius's house, he began to tell them about Jesus. He preached the Word to them, and they responded:

> While Peter was still speaking these words, the Holy Spirit came on all who heard the message. The circumcised believers who had come with Peter were astonished that the gift of the Holy Spirit had been poured out even on the Gentiles. For they heard them speaking in tongues and praising God.
>
> —Acts 10:44–46, NIV

Here not only is the gift of tongues mentioned, but we also see that the Holy Spirit is given only by faith, not by works or the Jewish law but by the hearing of the gospel.

Then six years after Pentecost, Paul found several disciples in Ephesus. Suspecting that something was missing there, he asked, "Did you receive the Holy Spirit when you believed?" (Acts 19:2, NIV). Paul was inquiring if, after salvation, they had received the baptism with the Holy Spirit. He recognized that there could be a delay, otherwise he would have asked if they were saved. "No," they said, "we have not even heard whether there is a Holy Spirit" (Acts 19:2, NASB).

As Paul questioned them further, he found out that they did not even know about Jesus, so he led them to accept Jesus as their Savior, and then they were baptized with water. (See Acts 19:4.). Later in Acts, we read, "Then, when Paul laid his hands upon their heads, the Holy Spirit came on them, and they spoke in other languages and prophesied. The men involved were about twelve in number" (Acts 19:6–7, TLB).

As I began to study the book of Acts, I realized that I, too, had been baptized in the Holy Spirit as a little girl. Twenty-five years later I understood what took place that day; the Lord baptized me in the Holy Spirit. Wow!

The early church was without doubt a praying church, and what tremendous things they accomplished through prayer alone: prison doors were opened, signs and wonders were done, and many people were added to the church. The early church was a praying church because they were filled with the Holy Spirit; and because they were filled, they prayed!

There will be times in each of our lives when we will not know how to pray effectively, but "the Spirit Himself intercedes for us with groaning too deep for words; and He who searches the hearts knows what the mind of the Spirit is, because He intercedes for the saints according to the will of God" (Rom. 8:27, NASB).

One day as I was sitting in a David Wilkerson rally intently listening to his sermon, I noticed after about ten minutes that I was quietly praying under my breath in tongues while listening to the Word. When I noticed what I was doing, I stopped. Then that still small voice within me said, "Do not stop, but intercede for souls."

What a fantastic opportunity to pray for people you do not even know! I personally would not have known how to pray for them as I should, particularly for an entire hour. God alone knows the need, and He communicates by His Spirit to our spirit how to pray in His perfect will. I always wondered how many believers God moved on to pray while David Wilkerson gave the message, but I do know that six thousand young people came forward that night. They wanted to be born again or set free from drugs, alcohol, or cigarettes. What a great opportunity to pray anytime during the day, as the Lord brings to your attention someone who needs prayer. There were many times, and still are, that I do not know how to pray. I do not always know the person's circumstances for whom I pray, but God does. There were times that I did not know how to pray for our son Simon, and all I could do was pray in the Spirit, trusting God to perfect my prayers.

It was but two months after the David Wilkerson rally that my husband came home from work one evening and said, "At, you will never believe what happened to me today at work."

"What?" I asked.

"I was in my office and I felt the presence of God all around me. I began to worship the Lord and put my hands up, and the Lord filled me with His Spirit. I received the baptism in the Holy Spirit, right at work!" Both of us smiled and thanked the Lord.

For God is at work within you, helping you want to obey him, and then helping you do what he wants.

—Philippians 2:13, TLB

7

A STRUGGLE

Every month we attended the Kathryn Kuhlman service. Many people were born again, healed of a wide variety of diseases, and set free from alcohol or drugs. It was an inspiration to all of us to see the power of God at work.

What I learned from Miss Kuhlman was that "with God, nothing is impossible." She always gave God all the glory and honor due Him. She truly was a woman of the Lord.

Seeing so many people set free, we thanked God, knowing what it meant to them. When they laughed, we laughed; when they cried, we cried. Looking at my little son's face next to me, I would pray, "Oh, Lord, heal him, too." When I did not see any change, I became frustrated and bewildered.

I thought perhaps God did not love me or maybe I had done something wrong; otherwise, He would heal Simon. For some inexplicable reason, I had a strange idea that God only healed those He loved. I was sadly mistaken and had a distorted perception of the love God has for us. His love is perfect, not at all like our love.

We sometimes equate love with getting what we want, but that can be the most selfish kind of love. Perfect love thinks about others and handles situations according to what is best for them. Perfect love sees further than today.

I thought my overriding need was healing for Simon, and then everything would be fine. But God knew there was a deeper need in my life, and this could be fulfilled when I surrendered my will to Him. God looked at the total picture. He knew nothing would be solved in my life if He gave me what I wanted, when I wanted it. I was yet to understand how great His love was for us. David knew about it when he wrote:

> O Lord, you have examined my heart and know everything about me. You know when I sit or stand. When far away you know my every thought. You chart the path ahead of me, and tell me where to stop and rest. Every moment you know where I am. You know what I am going to say before I even say it.
>
> —Psalm 139:1–4, TLB

Every week I went to a Bible study, and every time I went, it was as if the Lord spoke to me personally. One day it was on obeying God. We had to read a book called *The School of Obedience*. I loved that book. I learned that obedience is not just a single act but a life principle. Jesus said, "I do not seek My own will but the will of the Father who sent Me" (John 5:30). He lived and carried out the will of God, "Not My will, but Yours, be done" (Luke 22:42). Wow! And He is willing to make it so in us. That is what He promised when He said, "For whosoever shall do the will of God, the same is my brother, and my sister, and mother" (Mark 3:35, KJV).

As I was reading my Bible the next day, I distinctly knew that this is what I wanted. I wanted to do what the Lord wanted me to do, though I did not know how. I really had to think about it. Obedience to God is dying to the self. It is an emptying of self and letting God be God, a total surrender to Him. I did not know where to start. "How, God?" I wondered. "How can I die to self?" Then I began to understand as I had what I call a divine revelation. The Holy Spirit was so kind. He allowed me to experience, just for a second, what it was like to experience being totally yielded to God and to let God be God—all of Him and nothing of me. It became clear to me that I no longer had any say about my life, and I said to the Lord, "But God, then I have nothing to say any more but, 'Not I, but Christ in me.'"

"Yes," the Lord said, "is that what you want?"

I took but a second to respond. "Yes," I replied. "This is what I want."

When we make this statement of faith, the Holy Spirit begins His work in us:

> I have been crucified with Christ; it is no longer I who live, but Christ lives in me; and the life which I now live in the flesh I live by faith in the Son of God, who loved me and gave Himself for me.
>
> —Galatians 2:20

I began to understand that the Lord will work His nature in me, and I will work it out in obedience to the Lord. Obedience to God is so important. It means "not My will, but Yours, be done" (Luke 22:42). I was afraid of what would happen if God's will were not my will! I wanted Simon healed. "What if the Lord said no?" I wondered. Jesus, in the Garden of Gethsemane, prayed this prayer at a most crucial time of His life:

> And being found in appearance as a man, He humbled Himself and became obedient to the point of death, even the death of the cross.
>
> —Philippians 2:8

Even though Jesus was God's Son, He learned from experience what it was like to obey, even when obeying meant suffering.

> And having been made perfect, He became to all those who obey Him the source of eternal salvation.
>
> —Hebrews 5:9, NASU

"Sure," I reasoned, "Jesus is the Son of God. But what about the scripture that says He 'healed all who were ill?'"[14] I wondered. God's Word teaches us that it is the will of God to heal. So how could I then say, Your will be done? I was utterly confused. What I did not understand was that the Lord was dealing with me on the basis of His will being done. First things first; you have to have a solid foundation to build on. You cannot build your house on quicksand, for when the rains and floods come, the house will collapse. The wise man will build his house on the solid rock, and it will stand firm in the time of a storm—and we all will experience the storms of life. (See Matthew 7:24–25, NASU.) When that time comes, we better have a solid foundation to stand on. I did not have that solid foundation. I had to start from scratch. I wanted a healing, then all my problems would be solved.

"No," the Lord said. "You need to trust Me. You need to turn everything over to Me, and I will decide what is the best for everyone's life, including yours. Trust Me!"

I could not comprehend this. I was Simon's mom; I knew what Simon needed, and he needed a healing! But then this verse came up over and over again in my mind: "Not My will, but Yours, be done" (Luke 22:42).

There were times when my husband and I came home from church, encouraged to claim a healing. But then doubts began to emerge and I would say to Simen, "Tell me one more time, what does it really mean, 'Not My will, but Yours, be done'?" He would ask, "Do you believe it was the Lord who gave us the book *I Believe in Miracles* through your mom, Attie?"

"Yes," I said.

"Okay," my husband said. "Do you also believe it was no coincidence that we saw the program *I Believe in Miracles* that Sunday evening?" I agreed that it was not a coincidence, but a

14. Matt. 8:16, NASB

miracle. "Well then," my husband said, "I believe God is going to do something. Simon is going to get healed."

I looked at him and asked Simen, "How can you be so sure?"

"Think, Attie," he said, "why would God send us to a healing service and not heal Simon? I do not think so!" he said. "Let's believe the Lord. For I believe these incidents were no coincidences—they were God-incidents!" he continued. "Attie, you have to look at this the right way, from the Lord's standpoint. Why not give Simon over to the Lord and see what God is going to do?" Simen asked me.

"Yes," I said, "it makes sense as we go over the last couple of months, how the Lord has led us. But I cannot get away from the Bible verse that says, 'Not My will, but Yours, be done.'"

"Well," Simen said, "then give Simon over to the Lord, Attie."

"But how can I give him over to the Lord? I have tried it, and I am still worried. I do not know how I can give him over to the Lord and leave him there! I do not even know if I really want to. What is God going to do when I do that?" I pleaded.

My husband was listening to me as I rambled on. Finally he said, "Let's bring it to the Lord in prayer and ask Him to help us. It makes no sense to me that the Lord is leading us to a miracle service and not going to heal Simon. I am sure He is!"

"Yes," I said. I had to agree it made sense.

Sometimes as you look back on your life, you can clearly see the hand of the Lord guiding you, but when you are going through it, it is difficult to recognize the Lord in it until later. And then you realize the Lord was present, and you are in awe.

I read a similar story in Judges 13:2–24 where we see a couple, Manoah and his wife, wanting a child. Then one day the Angel of the Lord appeared to the wife saying, "Even though you have been barren for so long, you will conceive and have a son!" Then the Angel gave instruction for her special son—what to feed him and never to cut his hair. This child would be a special child, a Nazirite, dedicated to God.

> This child was called "Samson." Most of us have heard the story of Samson, the strong man with the long hair, but I had never thought about how he was conceived, who his parents were, or what the story about his birth was. It was quite a remarkable story, if you think about it. The Lord gave the mother special instructions on how to bring up her son. So when her husband came home, she shared what just took place. "We are going to have a baby!" she said.
>
> "Then Manoah prayed and asked God, Please let this man of God come back to us again, and give us more instructions about the baby you are going to give us." He believed his wife, and above all he believed the Lord. God answered his prayer, and the Angel of the Lord appeared once again to his wife as she was sitting in the field. She told the Angel, "Wait, I will get my husband because he wants to talk to you." She quickly ran and found her husband and said, "Manoah, the man is back. Come!" Manoah ran back with his wife and asked, "Are you the man who talked to my wife the other day?"
>
> "Yes," the Angel replied, "I am."
>
> So Manoah asked him, "Can you give us any special instruction about how we should raise the baby after he is born?" Then the Angel told them how to raise their son, and after he finished giving them instructions, Manoah said, "You've got to stay with us and have something to eat."
>
> "I'll stay," the Angel said, "but I cannot eat anything."
>
> "Why not?" Manoah asked. "What is your name?"

> "Don't ask my name," the Angel replied, "for it is a secret."
>
> Then Manoah took a young goat and a grain offering and offered it as a sacrifice to the Lord; and the Angel did a strange and wonderful thing. For as the flames of the altar were leaping up toward the sky and as Manoah and his wife watched, the Angel ascended in the fire!
>
> Manoah and his wife fell face downward to the ground. It was then that Manoah finally realized that it had been the Angel of the Lord. And there is the point of the story.
>
> "We will die," Manoah cried out to his wife, "for we have seen God!"
>
> "No," his wife said. "If the Lord were going to kill us He wouldn't have accepted our burnt offerings and wouldn't have appeared to us and told us these wonderful things and done these miracles!" Manoah's wife looked back, even though she did not understand it all, but she believed the Lord.
>
> —Author's paraphrase

What a story, and so it is with us. Looking back can bring us to see things more clearly. It makes us think that God is in this place and that place, and He is leading us this far, and He will lead us where we need to go. "And when their son was born they named him Samson."

And I am sure that God who began the good work within you will keep right on helping you grow in his grace until his task within you is finally finished on that day when Jesus Christ returns.

—Philippians 1:6, TLB

8

TOTAL SURRENDER

Several times a week, Simon and I went for physical therapy. In that time we got to know the therapist very well. One particular day there seemed to be something bothering her, and I asked her what it was.

"Well," she said, "we have to start thinking of how to best train Simon."

"Train Simon," I asked. "Why?"

"Simon is not making the progress I had hoped for," she said. "It is up to you and Simon to think of how he will spend the rest of his life, because he will get progressively stiffer throughout his body. We must decide the course of his therapy by training his body in a reclining or sitting position," she said.

I was horrified listening to her, and responded angrily, "No way! God is going to heal Simon!"

She paused for a moment, looked at me intently, and said, "Sit down for a moment, Mrs. De Vries." I made an attempt to leave, fighting back tears, and then I sat down. I assumed she thought I needed to face reality.

Her face was kind as she spoke. "I want to share something with you," she said gently, sensing how painful this conversation was for me.

"First of all," she began, "I have noticed that children who have parents who pray do much better than other children." Then she proceeded to tell me that Simon reminded her of her brother, and I knew that was why she liked him. "I also had a sister," she continued, "who, at the age of five, was a very sick little girl. Her fever was extremely high for days. My mother prayed for healing, just pleading with God to let her live. It was a miracle that my sister lived as long as she did, because my mother held on to her, not able to let her daughter go, until one day when she prayed, 'God, not my will, but Your will be done!' That moment she gave her little girl to the Lord, and my sister went to be with Jesus," the therapist continued. "My mother, in relinquishing her daughter to the Lord, experienced the peace of God. God was waiting all that time for my mother to release her little girl to Him and to trust God."

I listened to her, and as I drove home I was very upset. I cried and I cried, saying to myself, "I will never give Simon to God. What if He takes Simon home? No way!"

Simon, sitting next to me in the car, saw my tears and thought I was tired from driving. He looked up to me and said, "Mom, we can live close to the hospital so you won't be tired anymore!"

"It is all right, Simon," I said. I hugged him and we laughed.

Simon never heard the conversation between the therapist and me, but I could not forget what she had shared with me. She had quoted the very scripture and verse that had bothered me for months. Would I ever be able to surrender Simon to God? No, never. I would quote more positive scriptures, such as, "Ask whatever you wish, and it shall be done for you,"[15] or "He sent His Word and healed them."[16]

There was nothing wrong with those scriptures, except God had not given them to me.

I had presumed something God had never spoken to me. But God has ways of bringing us to that moment in our lives when, by His grace and the help of the Holy Spirit, we are able to say, "Your will be done." It is not in our strength, but by His, that we are able to surrender all.

15. John 15:7, NAS
16. Psalm 107:20, NAS

As I was driving to the hospital, I turned on the radio to hear a minister say, "Maybe you have questions such as, Why did this or that have to happen to me?" He went on to explain that in life it is as if someone had given you a piece of butter to eat by itself; you would not like it. Then he continued, "If I had to eat a cup of flour and a little bit of salt—it would be awful! And if you are like me and do not care for milk, but you had to drink a cup, that would not be so pleasant, either. But then you eat some sugar, which would be all right. Then you mix the butter, flour, salt, milk, and sugar together and put it in the oven for about one hour. And what comes out? A beautiful cake! That is how it is in life's experiences," the radio minister concluded. I smiled when I heard that.

When we arrived at the hospital for our next appointment, I was not aware that this day was to be the beginning of a very difficult decision we would be facing soon. After the doctor examined Simon, he suggested that we consider a new drug, also used on some cancer patients. Simon's condition was not improving, but getting worse at a steady pace. There was no guarantee that the drug would help, but there seemed no other choice. In order for them to administer this new drug, he said, "I want first to do some blood tests on Simon, which can be done this afternoon, and we should have all the results in by next week. So let us make another appointment for three weeks from today, December 18."

"What are the side effects of this new drug, doctor?" I asked.

"There is a danger that his white blood cells will greatly be reduced, making him susceptible to a life-threatening infection," the doctor explained. "And that is why I would like to wait a few weeks, to see how Simon is doing. If there is no improvement in his condition, you might consider this new drug. Because of the possible side effects, you and your husband have to sign a release for the hospital and doctors to administer this drug."

"What are we going to do?" I thought. "What is God's will in all of this?" I wondered. I felt a heavy load on myself as I drove home. Explaining to my husband what the doctor had told me, I said, "Simen, what shall we do?"

"Let's just wait and see," Simen replied. "Maybe God will let us know."

Everyone I asked said, "Attie, it is up to you and Simen. Pray about it." I was torn about what the right answer was. "What if we gave Simon the drugs and something happened to him?" I kept worrying. It would be our fault! I never have prayed so much in my life. I was continually pleading with God, literally "praying without ceasing." (See 1 Thessalonians 5:17.) I was determined not to give up until the answer came. "What do you want me to do, God? Should we give Simon the medicine?" I prayed. Looking back on all this, I know that even though I did not say it, I hoped every time we visited the doctor he would have a cure, or at least I looked to the doctor for some kind of hope. And this time I realized he was as dependent as I was on God's help, only he was not a believer and I was. That day, it felt as if there was no help; even the doctors did not know what to do or say. Only the Lord could help us.

I was at the lowest point of my life when I realized it was only God and me, and Simen, and Simon. No one else could help us. It was as if my back and Simon's were against the wall and there was nowhere to go but to God. And in the quietness of our bedroom, I knelt down and cried out to God. I felt the overwhelming love of God all around me, when God spoke to my heart and said, "Why are you so afraid to give Simon over to Me?"

"Well," I responded, "You might take him home."

"What is so bad to be with Me in heaven?"

It made me stop and think for a minute. If we say we love God, why are we then so reluctant to go to heaven? Then this still small voice said, "I love him far more than you will ever love him!" God, in a split second, let me feel the love He had for Simon. I felt the love of God all around me, and I realized that the way I look at Simon was the way God looked at me. More than anything, God wanted me to trust Him. For the first time in all those months, I understood. I knew. I felt the overwhelming love of God.

It was then that I was able to give Simon over to God. I said, "God, here is Simon. I give him to You. Not my will, but Yours be done. At that very moment I released him to the Lord. Absolute peace went through me. Everything became still inside of me. All the turmoil left. It was as if something had fallen off me, and I felt free. I knew that night that whatever God would decide was for our good.

The Lord brought me to the place of surrender so that His will could be done in my life and in the life of our son. No more taking him back—just leaving him with the Lord and simply trusting the Lord and resting in Him. With it came such inner peace.

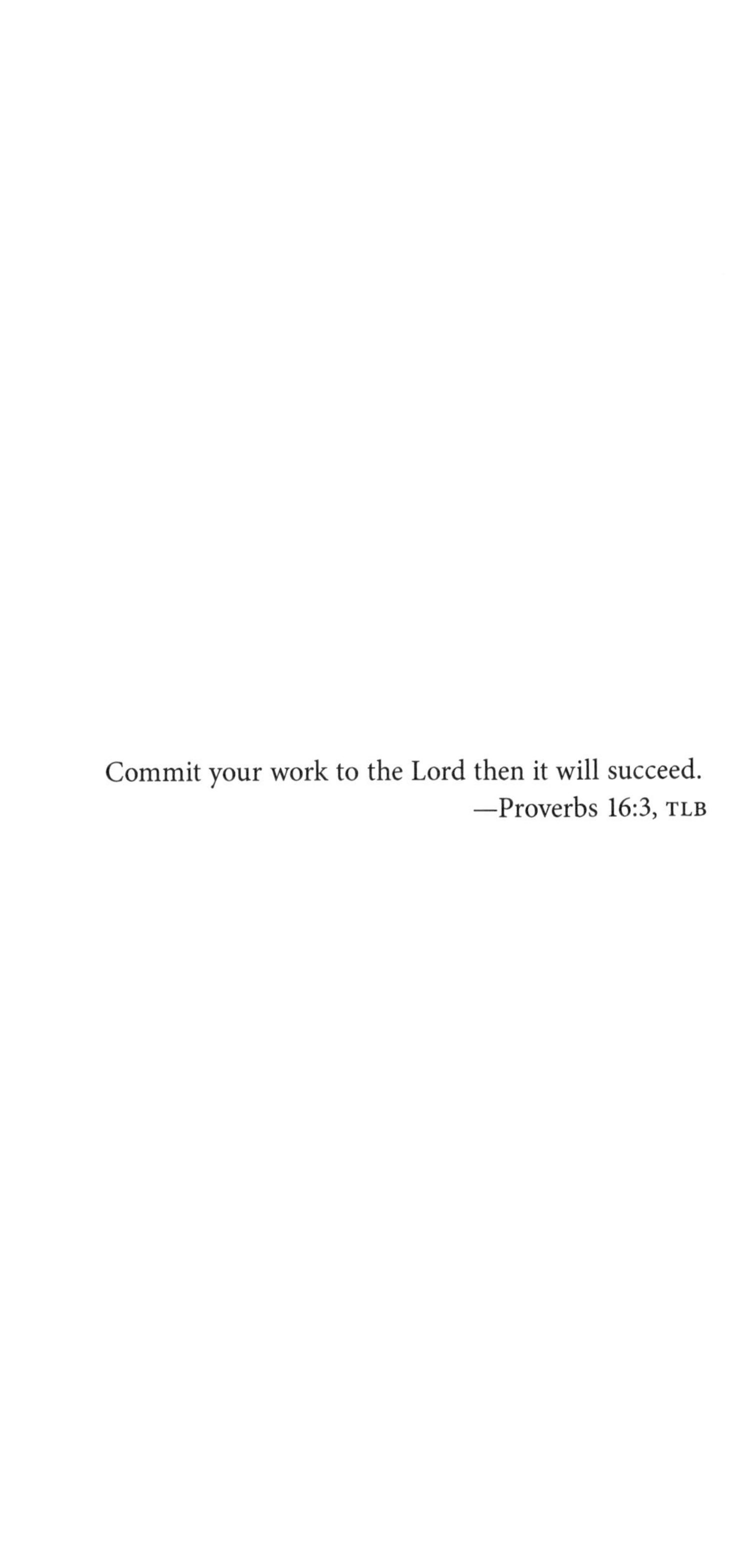

Commit your work to the Lord then it will succeed.
—Proverbs 16:3, TLB

9

THE PEACE OF GOD

THE NEXT MORNING I woke up a different person. The sun was coming through the bedroom window, and I enjoyed every minute of it. I lay there quietly, peaceful. This had not happened for months. There was such tranquility, peace, closeness with the Lord; I felt a deep peacefulness I had not felt in a long time. I used to wake up with terrible thoughts that something was wrong, and then I would remember, "Oh, yes, Simon is sick!" Then a feeling of panic would hit me, weighing me down the rest of the day. That next morning was different.

It was a beautiful morning. I knew God was going to see us through, and that the Lord had revealed Himself to me the night before, as I surrendered our son to Him. The peace I felt in my heart did not leave. It was wonderful. Our world was not perfect; Simon was still sick, yet I had a deep abiding peace in my heart.

In the Bible, there are two kinds of peace described. First, when we are born again, we have peace with God. The Amplified Bible says it like this:

> Therefore since we are justified (acquitted, declared righteous, and given a right standing with God) through faith, let us [grasp the fact that we] have [the peace of reconciliation to hold and to enjoy] peace with God through our Lord Jesus Christ (the Messiah, the Anointed One).
>
> —Romans 5:1, AMP

This peace you experience immediately as you become a child of God.

The second peace we are talking about is when you surrender your will to God and trust Him. No matter what takes place in our lives—a sick child, a money problem, the death of a loved one—we may cry, but there will be an abiding peace in our heart. The apostle Paul says it like this:

> Do not fret or have any anxiety about anything, but in every circumstance and in everything, by prayer and petition (definite requests), with thanksgiving, continue to make your wants known to God. And God's peace [shall be yours, that tranquil state of a soul assured of its salvation through Christ, and so fearing nothing from God and being content with its earthly lot of whatever sort that is, that peace] which transcends all understanding shall garrison and mount guard over your hearts and minds in Christ Jesus.
>
> —Philippians 4:6–7, AMP

This is the same Paul whose life was totally transformed on the road to Damascus when Jesus entered his heart and changed him from one of the fiercest opponents of the gospel to one of greatest defenders of Christ. He also said he had learned:

> How to be abased and live humbly in straitened circumstances, and I know also how to enjoy plenty and live in abundance. I have learned in any and all circumstances the secret of facing every situation, whether well-fed or going hungry, having a sufficiency and enough to spare or going without and being in want.
>
> —Philippians 4:12, AMP

The apostle Paul had learned the secret of not only giving his life over to God, but also trusting the Lord in everything, to totally surrender His life to the Lord. He was sold out to God.

As I read the Scriptures, especially the book of Acts, I marvel at what the disciples went through and their faith in God, even though they had a lot of opposition to the gospel being preached. Paul was put in jail and suffered a shipwreck, yet he trusted God when he was on the sea and a big storm came. There are times that we find ourselves in the storms of life. Paul began to seek the Lord, and an angel of the Lord said to him, "'Do not be afraid, Paul; you must be brought before Caesar; and indeed God has granted you all those who sail with you.' Therefore take heart, men, for I believe God that it will be just as it was told me" (Acts 27:24–25). I have known the Scriptures and have read them, believed them, yet failed to put them into practice.

You cannot simply have the peace of God because you have heard a lot. Read the Bible and expect to have the peace of God in your innermost being, which only comes by doing the will of God. If I neglect to acknowledge God as Lord of my life, with all its struggles, turmoil, and trials, I will lose the peace of God in my heart.

> Those things, which ye have both learned, and received, and heard, and seen in me, do: and the God of peace shall be with you.
>
> —Philippians 4:9, KJV

> Let the peace of God rule your hearts.
>
> —Colossians 3:15, KJV

It was not until some weeks later that I understood even better what miracle had taken place in my inner being. It was quiet and everyone was asleep when Simon woke up in pain. As I explained in an earlier chapter, fluid would build up between his joints and the pain was severe. What relieved it for a little while was a hot bath. Simon would then be able to fall asleep. An hour later, Simon would wake up again, and I would give him another hot bath. Sometimes I had to do this three or four times a night. I would feel so sad for him to see him in so much pain. I still did that particular evening, but it was different; there was peace in my heart. I had to pinch myself and ask, "Am I the same person, so calm and peaceful?" Wow! That was all I could say. That was not me. It was a work of God.

Again, I saw this principle of trusting God and releasing to the Lord whatever it is we are asking for demonstrated in our son Michael's life. A local minister at our church shared one evening how the Lord had answered the prayers of his son, whose bike had been stolen. Michael listened intently because his bike also had been stolen the day before. Coming home he announced, "I am asking the Lord to bring my bike back, for He knows where it is." He was six years old at the time. For the next six weeks he prayed earnestly, believing that God would return his bicycle.

After about one week, Michael's prayer changed. He was now more interested in the boy who stole the bike. (He was sure it was a boy.) "God, will you please give the boy who stole my bike a Bible for Christmas?" he prayed. And every evening he would thank the Lord for bringing the bike back and for the boy who stole it.

In the meantime, God set into motion a series of incidents. We needed a lawn mower, so when we drove home one Sunday, my husband noticed a sign on the front lawn of a house. It read, "Power lawn mower for sale." He stopped the car and went to the house, asking the man to keep the lawn mower for him until the next day.

"Sure," the man said. "I'll put it in the backyard for you until tomorrow." The next day as we all sat around the dinner table, Michael again prayed, "Thank you, Jesus, for bringing back my bike." By this time six weeks had passed, but there was no bike yet.

My husband looked at me and said, "God had better do something." Our faith had started to waiver, but not Michael's. After dinner my husband said, "Who is going with me for the lawnmower?"

"Me, Dad!" Michael said, and away they went, not knowing what was in store for them. When they arrived at the man's house, he told them to go with him into the backyard. There, Michael's eyes opened wide. "My bike!" he said. "That's my bike!"

The man had found the bike weeks ago in the river behind his house. He had fixed and cleaned it because, he said, "I felt someone would come for it."

We all learned a valuable lesson from the way our son prayed. First, he really wanted his bicycle back. After a while, he released it and became more concerned for the boy who stole it. The bike took second place. Then the Lord gave him the assurance that his bike would be found. Michael did not hold on to the bike, and in releasing it, God answered his prayer.

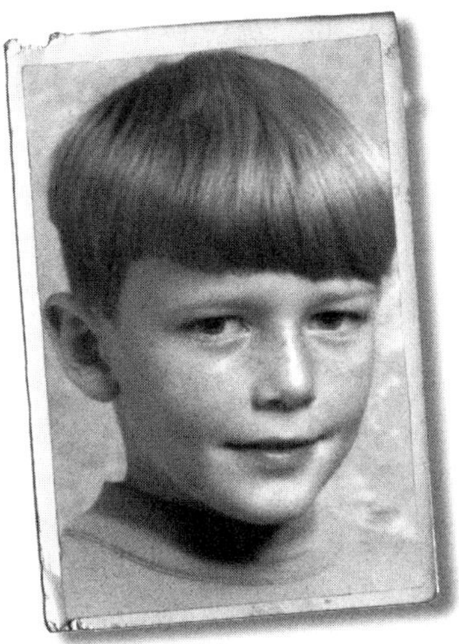

Michael

The best thing today that we can do for ourselves is—yes, that's right!—give everything over to the Lord, starting with ourselves, our children, our spouse, our work, and our finances. Everything!

But they that wait upon the Lord shall renew their strength. They shall mount up with wings like eagles; they shall run and not be weary; they shall walk and not faint.

—Isaiah 40:31, TLB

10

WAITING ON GOD

I FINALLY REALIZED HOW dependent I was on the Lord, even in how to pray. "Lord," I asked, "what do you want me to pray for next?" With this turnabout in my prayer life, something took place in my spirit, and faith began to grow.

"Is Simon going to get healed?" I asked. "God, is this from you?" I did not want to make the same mistake again of presuming something God had never said. So I was careful, waiting on the Lord for every answer. But a quiet knowing in my spirit started to grow; an assurance that God was going to heal Simon.

Joy welled up from deep within. It was as if God had said, "Yes, I am going to heal Simon. Let me work things out My way, for My timing is perfect." Or better yet:

> This plan of mine is not what you would work out, neither are my thoughts the same as yours! For just as the heavens are higher than the earth, so are my ways higher than yours, and my thoughts than yours. As the rain and snow come down from heaven and stay upon the ground to water the earth, and cause the grain to grow and to produce seed for the farmer and bread for the hungry, so also is my Word. I send it out, and it always produces fruit. It shall accomplish all I want it to and prosper everywhere I send it.
>
> —Isaiah 55:8–11, TLB

Then God told me, "Just follow what I am doing and pray accordingly." I finally began to understand it and literally ceased from doing anything and waited on the Lord. It was as if the Lord said, "You had better take a rest. You prayed hard and long enough in your own strength."

Paul E. Billheimer, in his book *Destined for the Throne*, an excellent book on prayer, says, "Prayer is not overcoming reluctance in God. It is not persuading Him to do something He is unwilling to do. It is binding upon Earth that which 'is already bound in heaven' (Matt. 16:19, AMP)." Billheimer continues, "It is implementing His decision. It is enforcing His will upon the Earth. Prayer makes possible God's accomplishing what He wants, and He cannot do without our prayers. The content of all true prayer originates in the heart of God, so it is He who inspires prayer in the hearts of man. The answer to every God-inspired petition is already prepared before the prayer is uttered."[17]

When we understand this, faith is simple. It is not us but God we have to look to, for He is the author and the finisher of our faith. (See Hebrews 12:2.) We can never please God without faith, without depending on Him. Anyone who wants to come to God must believe that there is a God and that He rewards those who sincerely look for Him. (See Hebrews 11:6.)

During this period I also became more aware of the Lord ministering to my spirit. The Word says that "the spirit of man is the lamp of the LORD, searching all the innermost parts of his being" (Prov. 20:27, NASB). It is the Spirit of God who teaches and communicates to our spirit the deep things of God. It is through the Holy Spirit that God unfolds His mind to our spirit so we can discern the will of God.

One day some friends of ours stopped by to see us and they asked how Simon was doing. I replied, to my amazement, "The Lord is going to heal him!" I started to laugh. Looking at my

17. Paul E. Billheimer, *Destined for the Throne* (Fort Washington, PA: Christian Literature Crusade, Inc., 1975), 52.

husband, I said, "Simen, did you hear what I just said? The Lord is going to heal Simon!"

We all laughed with joy! That was the first time I had confessed what was in my heart, and when I spoke, we all felt the joy of the Lord. When I confessed Simon's healing, I knew in my spirit it was done. But then I began having second thoughts. The devil was saying, "How do you know?" and "Did God say he was healed?" Simon was still in pain. There was no evidence of any healing yet, at least, not to the eye, but only by that inner knowing. Paul said we are to "take captive every thought to make it obedient to Christ" (2 Cor. 10:5, NIV). Every time I confessed what I knew to be true, it was as if something took root in my spirit and understanding. Praise the Lord!

There are times in each of our lives when all we can do is to trust God, knowing that God is in control. Catherine Marshall wrote a book called *Something More*. It has a chapter that states, "Yes, God is in everything." That is a big statement, something to think about. "Is God in everything?" I wondered. "Do I believe this?" I asked myself. Or better yet, do *we* believe this? You can refute this and come up with many pros and cons. Romans 8:28 says, "All things work together for good to them that love God, to them who are the called according to His purpose" (KJV). Catherine Marshall states in her book that it took her twenty-seven years to finally acknowledge this.[18]

To know that God is in control and not me gave me an assurance and peace. For instance, when the decision had to be made whether Simon would take the experimental drug, I had not known what the Lord's will was. I had been afraid to give this medicine used on cancer patients to Simon because of its side effects. Now, I had peace of mind.

The Lord would decide whether Simon would get the drug or not. I knew only one thing—Simon was going to be healed God's way. How this was to be accomplished, I left to the Lord.

---

18. Catherine Marshall, *Something More* (New York: McGraw-Hill, 1974), 18.

Trusting the Lord

December 18, 1969, came and I prayed, "God, whatever Your will is in this matter, I will abide by it and I will co-operate with the doctors. But if Your will is not to give Simon this medicine, Lord, then let the doctors see some improvement in Simon's condition so the drug will not be necessary."

It was not the most perfect prayer, but it was all I knew. I felt it was out of my hands, and I knew God's will would be done. After the doctor examined Simon thoroughly, he looked at me and said, "Mrs. De Vries, I feel there is some improvement. Therefore I suggest we postpone giving Simon the medicine for another six weeks." Praise the Lord! I believed then Simon would never have the medicine, and he never did.

It was a miracle for the doctor to have said what he did, because I did not see any improvement in Simon. I believe there are times when we do not know how to pray, for the simple reason that God is saying, "Do you trust Me enough to leave it with Me? I will take care of this. Just trust Me!" It is easy to say, "Yes, God, I trust you," until we are faced with a difficult situation. How do we react to it? Do we have the peace of God? Only the Lord can give us this peace of mind, even in the midst of the most difficult situations.

Through all this we learn to depend on the Lord. There is a song written by Andraé Crouch that says it so well:

Through It All
by Andraé Crouch

I've had many tears and sorrows;
I've had questions for tomorrow;
There've been times I didn't know right from wrong;
But in ev'ry situation, God gave blessed consolation,
That my trials come to only make me strong.

Chorus:
Through it all,
Through it all,
Oh I've learned to trust in Jesus,
I've learned to trust in God.
Through it all,
Through it all,
Oh I've learned to depend upon His Word.

I've been to lots of places,
And I've seen a lot faces;
There've been times I felt so all alone;
But in my lonely hours, yes, those precious lonely hours,
Jesus let me know that I was His own.

I thank God for the mountains,
And I thank Him for the valleys;
I thank Him for the storms He brought me through;
For if I'd never had a problem,
I wouldn't know that He could solve them,
I'd never know what faith in God could do. [19]

Discerning What to Pray For

Simon was still not free from pain, but after two weeks I noticed a slight improvement. The pain was not as severe and did not last quite as long. Every few weeks Simon developed an infection in both hips, resulting in intense pain and preventing him from walking. Usually this lasted about three days. Knowing the Lord was doing something, I prayed accordingly.

The next Kathryn Kuhlman service came, and my husband and I went. Simon was unable to go because of pain, so we decided

19. © Copyright 1971. Renewed 1999 by Manna Music, Inc., 35255 Brooten Road, Pacific City, OR 97135. All Rights Reserved. Used by Permission. (ASCAP)

"Well," she explained, "around three o'clock, Simon got up from the couch and said, 'I feel good, Oma. May I go play outside? I have no pain anymore, Oma. It is gone, so can I play outside?'" My mother explained he was indeed feeling fine, so she told him, "Sure, go play with your friends."

"I watched him," she said, "and he is doing fine."

"Oh, Mom," I said, "God healed Simon. We prayed for him this afternoon, the same time you said he got up from the couch and said there was no more pain!" We all thanked the Lord for this miracle.

That day Simon was completely set free of pain and he began to improve. Many of our friends and relatives were praying, not only for Simon, but also for us as a family. Sharing this with our doctor, I asked him to give an evaluation of how he felt Simon was doing. His letter is shown on page 91.

We give God all the praise for this. And when we were given the opportunity to share what the Lord had done, we were more than thankful that the Lord let us share in the miracle. As we attended the miracle service, a lady who was Miss Kuhlman's close friend and worker approached us as we walked into the healing service. She asked, "How are you doing? How is Simon doing?"

As we shared with her what the Lord had done in our lives and how He had healed Simon, she asked if we would be willing to give our testimony on the television program *I Believe in Miracles*. This program aired every Sunday evening and was the same program that gave us encouragement in July of 1969. We felt it was a fantastic opportunity to tell millions of people that God is still on the throne and heals people. He healed Simon, and what He did for us, He will do for them!

My husband and Simon gave their testimony that day, September 29, 1971, as I sat in the audience praying. Many of our neighbors saw what the Lord had done in our lives. Whenever I had an opportunity, I shared with them. Also, our children played with the neighbor's children, and they all knew what God had done. So we decided after we prayed about it to have a neighborhood Bible study. Most of our neighbors came every Saturday evening. Many of them accepted the Lord. We saw many prayers answered, and if any of our neighbors needed prayer, they would come to our home and we all prayed.

CHILDRENS HOSPITAL OF LOS ANGELES

4650 SUNSET BOULEVARD · NORMANDY 3-3341 · MAILING ADDRESS: P.O. BOX 54700 · LOS ANGELES, CALIFORNIA 90054

March 25, 1971

Mrs. Simen DeVries
9020 Terhune Avenue
Sun Valley, California 91352

Dear Mrs. DeVries:

Until approximately last spring Simon suffered from a progressively severe scleroderma which affected the skin over most of his body and resulted in increasingly severe contractures of his fingers, knees, and hips. Since that time he has made steady improvement with the sclerodermatous skin lesions fading out and the motion of all his joints improving remarkably. The change represents a very marked improvement in his condition and has come about without the use of medication or other procedures such as surgical operations.

Sincerely yours,

Virgil Hanson

Virgil Hanson, M.D.
Associate Professor of Pediatrics
University of Southern California
School of Medicine

VH:ct

Great is his faithfulness; his lovingkindness begins afresh each day.

—Lamentations 3:23, TLB

11

GOD IS FAITHFUL

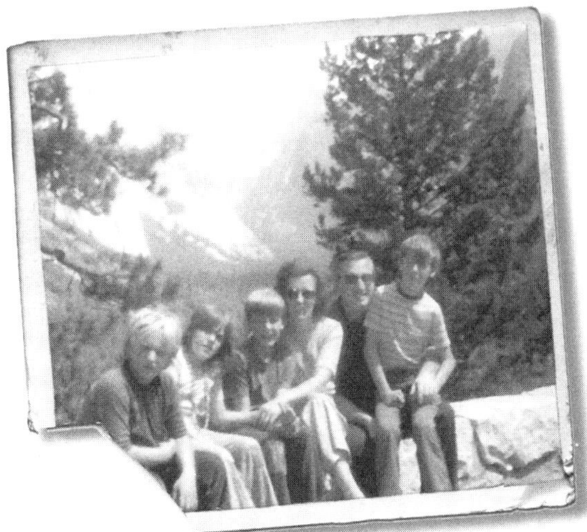

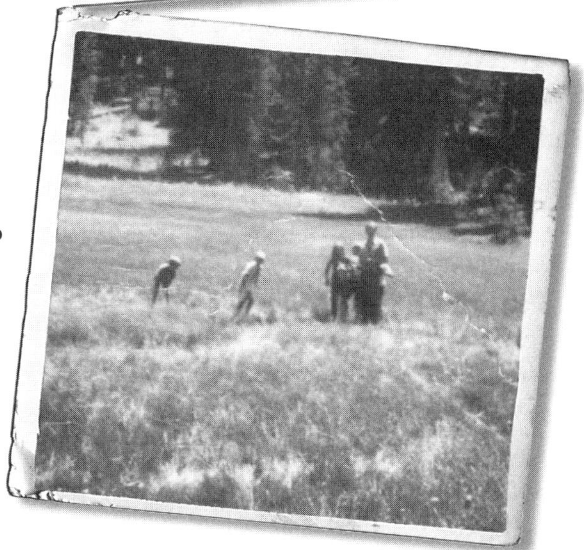

(above) Jo, Yvonne, Michael, Attie, Simen, and Simon

(R) Looking for the hubcap

Every summer we spent our vacation at Yosemite National Park. Yosemite Park was still a beautiful place to go camping, just as we had discovered a long time ago when we first got married. As you enter Yosemite Park, you see trees everywhere. You feel that you have just entered God's country, with all its beauty and majestic scenery. The winding road going up the mountains makes you wonder where it is going; it cannot be more beautiful! You see deer coming across the road, then you see the steeple of the Valley Church, and you know you have arrived!

I have never seen the sun shining so brightly, the sky so blue, as when we drive into Yosemite Park. It reminds me of Psalm 19:1–5 (TLB):

> The heavens are telling the glory of God; they are a marvelous display of his craftsmanship. Day and night they keep on telling about God. Without a sound or word, silent in the skies, their message reaches out to all the world. The sun lives in the heavens where God placed it and moves out across the skies.

It is truly God's country, a place you could live forever. I sometimes wonder if heaven is anything like this. Our family has grown since that first visit when I found out I was pregnant with our first baby. We now go with all four of our children, their friends, my brother and sister, and their families. It is a time of catching up for all of us and just relaxing together as a family.

As we were driving into the valley in our Lark Studebaker, the roof loaded with camping gear, we noticed we had lost one of our wheel covers. It came off and rolled into the high prairie grass in front of Camp Curry. We did not want to stop to get the wheel cover. Instead I said, "We will go back later to find it." As we entered our campground at North Pines, we found our usual spot by the river. We love to go to the same spot every year. It is a tradition. Simen and the boys set up the tent, while the girls helped me arrange the sleeping and cooking situation and decided where the table should go.

After we had everything set up, Simen asked, "Who will go with me to look for the hubcap?" They all wanted to go. After sitting in that car for ten hours and then setting up camp, they were ready to go for a ride. Also Rita, one of our cousins, went, leaving me at the campsite to fix dinner.

Dinner was almost ready when everyone arrived back at the camp. "Mom," Michael said, "You'll never guess what happened. We found the hubcap!"

"Really?" I asked.

"Yes, we all prayed," my husband said. They had literally combed that meadow slowly covering the whole area, but did not find the hubcap. Finally, Simen said, "You know what? God knows where it is. Why don't we just ask Him to let us know where it is?" They all held hands and prayed, simply asking God to show them where the hubcap was. As soon as they finished asking God to show them, they all ran to the same spot, almost bumping heads to pick up the hubcap. There it was, right in front of them. They all were surprised that it was so easy to find after they prayed.

It was a beautiful and powerful example of how the Lord answered their prayer. Even if it is only a hubcap, God wants us to talk to Him. Our children have never forgotten this, and neither have we.

After dinner we all sat around the campfire talking and sharing with the rest of the family, having a blessed time. When we all saw a bear coming right at our camp, we ran in the tents and of course made so much noise that the bear left. It was a day we never forgot, and we still talk about it when we are all together as a family.

The rivers at Yosemite are ice cold because the water comes from mountain snow. Simon had not been able to swim in such ice-cold water. But that summer of 1970, Simon asked, "Mom, can I go in the water? Please?"

"Sure," I said. "Have fun!"

This was a test for us, about how much we believed God. Simon was swimming with absolutely no pain; it was a miracle! We all thanked the Lord for what He had done. This was a big milestone in Simon's life, with no pain, playing with his brother, sisters, and cousins.

Every day we sat there by the river watching our children having fun. We all praised the Lord for what He had done. The Lord taught me to depend on Him in every circumstance.

We can miss God's dealings in our everyday lives by not being open to the Spirit of God. When reading the Word or when someone shares with us, we must always be discerning and say, "Is there something you want me to know, Lord?" Not everyone who comes to us is sent by God, for if it is not in accordance with the Word, we must ignore it. We test everything by Scripture!

There were many times someone shared with me about God, but I ignored it. Now the Lord gave me a second chance, and used people to speak to my heart. I learned a vital lesson that God uses whomever He wants, whenever He wants. Many a time someone ministered to me who probably was not aware of it. Our own children, as small as they were, have ministered to me. So all I am saying is this: be discerning.

Simon and I continued our usual routine of going three times a week for physical therapy. We shared with the therapist what the Lord had done, how Simon was able to swim in the cold water at Yosemite without pain.

She listened and said, "Why don't you ask the Lord for more strength for Simon so he can go to school full time?" (Simon was not able to go full time to school because of extreme tiredness.) Recognizing the Lord in this, I said, "Yes, I will." This was the same therapist who, some months prior, had shared with me the story of her sister's death and how her mother experienced the peace of God when she said, "Not my will, but Yours, be done." Simon continued going to school part time, and by September he was able to go for the full day, playing like any other child from early morning until it was time to go to bed.

In addition to Simon's scleroderma, he also had suffered from an enlarged liver and spleen. Due to the scleroderma, round nodules had formed along his spine. They were calcium deposits, the doctor explained. I prayed for the Lord to please heal his liver and spleen. During our next appointment I prayed, "Please, God, let the spleen and liver be back to normal." Every time the doctor checked his liver and spleen he would say, "They are both still enlarged." Also his blood test showed his SGOT was high, which indicates any form of abnormality in the liver or heart. He also had to have a liver biopsy, and all results were positive of scleroderma.

As we sat in the doctor's office, the doctor came in and asked, "Well, Simon, how are you today?" Simon always had something to share with the doctor, and as he did, the doctor examined his liver and spleen. I looked at him. "Well," I said, "how are his liver and spleen? Still enlarged?" He did not say anything and kept on examining Simon. Finally he said, "I will be right back." One by one, different doctors came in to check Simon.

"What are you looking for?" I asked. I noticed that they all checked Simon's arms, hands, fingers, and spine.

"Well," they explained, "the calcium deposits are gone." Simon had calcium deposits throughout his body, arms, fingers, and spine. I personally had observed that the nodules at his spinal cord had disappeared, but I did not know about his skin. Only the doctors could feel that, for it was deep in the skin. They were amazed that the calcium deposits were gone. As one doctor explained, "This never happens!"

Well, I said, "We prayed that God would heal Simon." One doctor responded by saying, "I am a believer, and I know God hears and answers our prayers."

The other doctors did not say anything. Our doctor, when he came back in, said to me, "Mrs. De Vries, not only are there no more calcium deposits, but his liver and spleen are back to normal." He looked at me, not knowing what else to say.

"We have asked God to heal Simon," I said.

"Maybe it is God, maybe not," he said. "I don't know." With that, he left the room.

That doctor was not a Christian, so it was difficult for him to respond. But going home, I sure was praising the Lord and thanking Him for what He had done! I realized I was getting a lesson in prayer, waiting on the Lord and seeing what He would want me to pray for and then see the prayer being answered. The Amplified Bible says, "And this is the confidence (the assurance, the privilege of boldness) which we have in Him: [we are sure] that if we ask anything (make any request) according to His will (in agreement with His own plan), He listens to and hears us. And if (since) we [positively] know that He listens to us in whatever we ask, we also know [with settled and absolute knowledge] that we have [granted us as our present possessions] the requests made of Him" (1 John 5:14–15).

There was one thing that still puzzled all of us. Simon's hands and feet were still deformed due to scar tissue. The therapist explained to me that wherever healing had taken place, scar tissue formed. There was nothing that could be done about it, except to continue the physical therapy in the hopes of preventing his hands and feet from becoming more deformed. But therapy was not going to stop it. All we could do was attempt to slow down the deterioration process. At this particular time, Simon's hands were staying pretty much at the same level, and the therapy at the hospital was discontinued. I knew Simon needed an instant miracle. My prayer was, "God, are you going to straighten his hands and feet, or are they going to stay the way they are?"

Then, one Thursday morning, as I attended a women's Bible study, I heard something that was of interest to me. The teacher said, "When God starts a healing, He will finish it, so don't stop praying too soon!" I knew this was for me; it made sense. Going home, I was determined to pray through. I believed God would answer and finish this healing.

I needed and appreciated the Word of God very much, and I respect teachers who are qualified to teach. Many times God has used them to speak a word of encouragement to me, a word I needed to hear right at that moment, or a Scripture verse I could stand on.

The Word of God

It was on a Monday morning in December 1974 when I was driving to school early in the morning, talking to the Lord, saying, "Lord, what do You want me to do? Should I continue the exercises with Simon? God, You promised a complete healing, and to me this is not complete, for Simon's hands are still deformed! Are You going to heal them, Lord?" At this time, I stopped the car to let two girls into the car to take them to school. All our children had been going to a private Christian school. Every Monday the children learn a Bible verse for school. Sitting right behind me, I overheard one of the girls say, "Ann, do you want to hear my Bible verse for today?" She then continued, "He staggered not at the promise of God through unbelief; but was strong in faith, giving glory to God; And being fully persuaded that, what he had promised, he was able also to perform." When she quoted that verse, I knew it was for me. "Ann," I asked, "where can I find that verse?" She responded, "Romans 4:20–21."[20]

I had just asked the Lord, Are you going to straighten Simon's hands completely, God? and the Lord gave me an answer. I was so thankful and praised the Lord for straightening Simon's hands before it happened. I believed what God promised, He would do.

---

20. KJV

I could not wait to get home to read the passage for myself. The moment I walked in the door, I opened my Bible to Romans 4:20–21 and began to read. But something strange took place. I did not recognize the verses. They did not seem like the same verses. Disappointed, I closed my Bible, not understanding what had just taken place. I turned on the radio to hear a minister conducting a daily Bible study.

"Today," he said, "we are going to read out of Romans, the fourth chapter." Excitedly I reached for my Bible. "Not the first half," he said, "but the second half." He then started to read, coming to the passage, "He [Abraham] staggered not at the promise of God through unbelief; but was strong in faith, giving glory to God; And being fully persuaded that, what he had promised, he was able also to perform" (Rom. 4:20–21, KJV). The Lord again quickened this verse to my heart. I knew it was for me. I had heard from the Lord.

Satan had tried to snatch away what was sown, but the Lord would always win out. In Matthew 13, Jesus explained what can happen when the Word is sown:

> He told them many things in parables [that is, stories by way of illustration], saying: "A farmer went out to sow his seed. As he was scattering the seed, some fell along the path, and the birds came and ate it up."
>
> —Matthew 13:3, NIV

This means that when someone hears the Word of God and does not understand it, Satan will come and take it away.

> Some fell on rocky places, where it did not have much soil. It sprang up quickly, because the soil was shallow. But when the sun came up, the plants were scorched, and they withered because they had no root.
>
> —Matthew 13:5–6, NIV

This man received the message with joy, but because of the rocky soil, he had areas in his life not yielded to God. This could mean earthly possessions, friends, or not putting God first in his life. And when persecution came, he gave up. His roots were not deep enough. But when our delight is in God, when we put Him fist in our lives, we will be "like a tree planted by streams of water" (Ps. 1:3, NIV).

> Other seeds fell among thorns, and the thorns choked out the tender blades.
>
> —Matthew 13:7, TLB

This man heard the message, but he also put money and the cares of this life before God. The result was that he drifted farther away from the Lord.

> But some fell on good soil and produced a crop that was thirty, sixty, and even a hundred times as much as he had planted.
>
> —Matthew 13:8, TLB

He not only heard the message, but responded to God and obeyed the Word.

But Abraham never doubted. He believed God, for his faith and trust grew ever stronger, and he praised God for this blessing even before it happened. He was completely sure that God was well able to do anything He promised.

—Romans 4:20–21, TLB

12

FAITH VS. FEAR

IT WOULD BE nice to say there were never any problems again, that I had learned everything there was to learn. But life is a process of continued learning and growing. We live by faith, and once we think we know how to conquer a problem, something else will take its place. Continued learning keeps us close to God.

One evening as all of us were asleep, Simon came to our bedroom. Waking up, I said, "Simon, what is it?"

"I am thirsty, Mom," he said. "Can I have something to drink?"

Looking at our son sitting across from our bed, my eyes were drawn to his hands. I noticed something strange. I saw that his hands had grown more closed. I was not expecting this.

"Simon," I said, "let me take a look at your hands." And as he put his small, deformed hands in mine, I was shocked! Why were they more crooked? I wanted to know. Fear struck me. I had never seen anyone healed and then lose their healing. I wondered, "Is there such an experience?"

"Simon," I asked, "when did your hands begin to grow more closed?"

"Oh, I do not know, Mom," he said. Simon had not paid any attention to it. God promised to straighten them and that settled it for him. All Simon was concerned about was his cup of milk.

I, too, had not paid attention to it. Simon did not have any pain, and we just left it all to God, until this evening. I had many questions, and after tucking Simon back into bed, I cried out to God, "Lord, why are his hands growing more closed? Why, God?" I was in a battle, and the devil was right there to snatch away the Word of God.

"Has God really said He would completely heal Simon?" the devil chided me. I began to wonder if it was really God who had told me. All the evidence was contrary to what the Lord had promised me! I believed God would straighten Simon's hands one day, but when I saw them growing more closed, I was not so sure. "How could this be?" I cried. "Do I still believe, when all evidence is in the opposite direction?" I wondered about myself. "Where in God's Word did it say that after He had given a promise to someone, He changed His mind? I do not know," I reasoned. "There are only two alternatives." I thought. "Either I am presuming, or God indeed did speak. I had better find out," I decided to myself. I began to feel a tremendous burden to pray. It was not a question of Simon's healing, for this had been settled when I gave Simon over to God. There was something more here.

For the next few weeks I prayed constantly, walking the floor back and forth for hours, praying in the Spirit, believing the Lord to perfect my prayers, and reading the Word of God to find out if God ever changed His mind by taking back a promise. I had to know. Not only was my faith tested, but I also began to realize the much deeper importance of knowing what God's Word said.

Every Wednesday evening I went to a Bible study at our church. The lesson that particular week was on Abraham and Isaac—how Abraham had grown strong in his faith, glorifying God, until finally, after twenty-five years, his promised son was born. I was encouraged that evening to stand fast, for it reaffirmed my faith that God's promises were always fulfilled.

Yet coming home and seeing my son's hands, I once again began to doubt. "Could I believe the Lord, even if all physical evidence was contrary to what God said would happen?" I wondered. "How could this be?" I asked myself.

The next day I took Simon to the doctor, and after his examination, the doctor said, "There is one thing we can do. The Arthritis Foundation does provide casts for children with arthritis. I suggest that we try this for Simon. Maybe he will benefit from it. We might prevent his hands from closing further." I made an appointment for the following day, and as I watched them build a cast around Simon's arms and wrists, it became a real test for me.

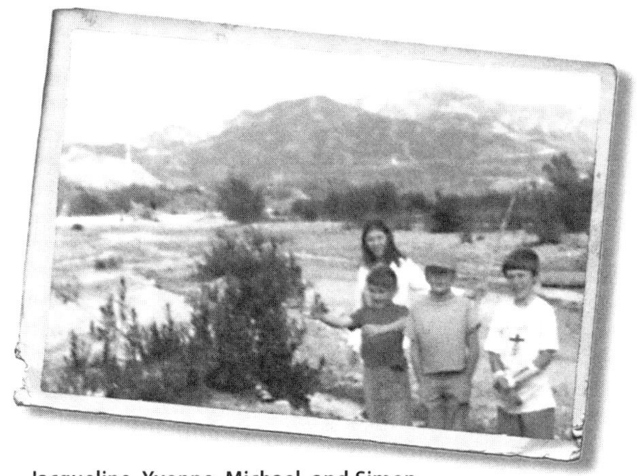

Jacqueline, Yvonne, Michael, and Simon

That evening Simon again woke up in an intense discomfort. The pressure of the cast produced pain around his wrist and fingers, so we cut some of the plaster loose to relieve the pressure. But some hours later Simon again woke up in pain. The next day we returned to the doctor and he decided to form another cast that might fit better. The same thing happened. Apparently Simon could not stand any pressure around his wrist and fingers, so this procedure was discontinued. We had done all we could for Simon.

A few weeks later I decided to attend another Wednesday Bible class. Once again the lesson was about Abraham and

Isaac. I began to wonder how this applied to me. I listened intently to the teacher as she explained that Abraham's story was not recorded for his benefit only, but for us also. (See Romans 4:23–24.)

Abraham was called the friend of God. (See James 2:23.) God made known His will over and over again to Abraham. What made this man so pleasing to God? Abraham believed that whatever God said, He would do. "By faith Abraham, when he was called, obeyed by going out to a place which he was to receive for an inheritance; and he went out, not knowing where he was going" (Heb. 11:8, NASB).

God also promised Abraham a son. Many years went by and still there was no son. So after he lived ten years in the land of Canaan, Abraham decided to give God a little help. (See Genesis 16:3.) He took Hagar the Egyptian to be his second wife. A son was born to them, and they called him Ishmael. God's plan was that Abraham would have a son fourteen years later by his wife Sarah, not by Hagar.

How many times do we also try to help God out and get in the way, instead of ceasing from all effort to patiently wait for the Lord's perfect timing? It was not that Abraham did not believe God, because we are told that, "Abraham believed the Lord; and he reckoned it to him as righteousness" (Gen. 15:6, RSV). But after waiting for so long and still no son, Abraham thought surely having a son with Hagar must be God's will, but he was mistaken. It was all his own doing, after the flesh. God told Abraham that his son would be born by Sarah, not Hagar. Isaac was the child God promised, a work of God's grace, meaning God working instead of Abraham. Everything we do and accomplish in our lives is meaningless if it is not of God.

The most difficult lesson we learn in life is to wait on God. That is why Paul said, "Hagar represents the Law—me working, instead of God. We are justified by faith, not by works!" (Gal. 2:16, author's paraphrase).

When the appointed time came for God to fulfill His promise to Abraham, he was one hundred years old and his body was as good as dead. (See Romans 4:19.) "For Sarah conceived and bore Abraham a son in his old age, at the set time of which God had spoken to him" (Gen. 21:2). Biologically, there would have been no way for Abraham and Sarah to have a son, but this was the time that God's power could be manifested. We, too, need to reckon ourselves dead so that we can believe in the God who gives life to the dead. Nothing is impossible with God. Many times the Lord waits until we cease from all labor and let Him take over. In waiting twenty-five years for Isaac to be born, Abraham learned a tremendous lesson in faith: "He staggered not at the promise of God through unbelief; but was strong in faith, giving glory to God; and being fully persuaded that, what he had promised, he was able also to perform" (Rom. 4:20, KJV).

Like Abraham, our faith, too, might be tried and tested. There may be times we want to give up. But we can't let ourselves be discouraged! God is faithful, and the very testing is the proof that God is preparing us for the blessing. I was encouraged, to say the least, but coming home was another story. Doubts started to emerge. I had many questions. I had to hear from God how this story applied to me personally.

We shared Simon's healing with all our neighbors. One neighbor asked me more than once, "Is Simon still healed?"

I wondered to myself, "What am I going to tell them? Would they still believe that the Lord healed when they saw Simon's hands? There is no way I can share this with them," I reasoned. They needed all the encouragement they could get. How could I have shared the truth that Simon's hands were still closing? And if I had shared that with them, would they have still believed that healing was for today, for them?" I remembered back to the time when it was so difficult for me to believe. And while I was washing the dishes, thinking about this, I said, "God, I don't understand what is going on. We shared with everyone that wanted to hear that You healed Simon, and now, God, it looks as if everything is wrong! Did I make a mistake, God? Did I do something wrong, God? I need to know. If I share this with our neighbors, will they still believe that You heal?"

I was pouring out my heart before the Lord when suddenly the Lord answered me and said, "It is not your ministry, but Mine!" Instantly I knew what I had done wrong. Whether Simon was healed or not was God's business. People would not believe just because Simon was healed. They would believe when God made it real to them. He was the One who gave the faith for this. What I was doing was defending the Word of God, and God's Word does not need any defense. Then the Lord spoke again, saying, "Would you be willing for Me to reverse the promise?" Then He also told me to trust Him.

"Yes, Lord," I said. I did not really know what it all meant. All I knew was that I had heard from the Lord. That is what I wanted to know—if God was still in all of this and if He knew about it. He did, and all was well.

Sometimes we have to give the promise back to God. Like death to a vision and to a promise, the Lord is saying, "Just trust Me. Give it all to Me."

You can fill in the rest of your questions: Why, God? What about…? God, what are You going to do, and why? And God is saying, "Just trust Me, I will work it out My way. Just look to Me."

In times like those, there will be nothing to hold on to but God! And that will be more than enough! The Lord does not want us not to hold on to even a promise, but only to Him! Abraham implicitly trusted God. Abraham, I am sure, did not understand everything, but He did trust the Lord. We know this because Abraham said to his young men, "Stay here with the donkey and I and the lad will go yonder; and we will worship and return to you" (Gen. 22:5, author's paraphrase). Notice the faith stated in the phrase, "I and the lad." No wonder he is called a friend of God.

Sharing with my husband that evening, he said, "You know, At, Abraham had to give Isaac to God." The whole three weeks, all I heard about was Abraham and Isaac. As I shared with my husband what had transpired that day, he said, "I also want what God wants, so let's pray together. God, we do not understand everything, but do whatever is pleasing to You. We give You back the promise of Simon's healing so that You might be glorified in this. Not our will be done, but Yours be done. Amen." The presence of God was all around us as we prayed together. We looked at each other with tears streaming down our faces, and we knew that the Lord was with us.

The next evening, Simen and I were sitting in the living room. Billy Graham was on television preaching about the verse, "The just shall live by faith" (Rom. 1:17). Once again, tears streamed down my face as I listened to how the Lord had tested the faith of Abraham.

> Now it came about after these things, that God tested Abraham, and said to him, "Abraham!" And he said, "Here I am." And He said, "Take now your son, your only son, whom you love, Isaac, and go to the land of Moriah; and offer him there as a burnt offering."
>
> —Genesis 22:1–2, NAS

God put Abraham to the supreme test so that all men might know that it was possible to love God more than anyone else. Abraham could have reasoned, "This cannot be the will of God. It must be a deception of the devil." Sacrificing Isaac would have meant sacrificing the covenant, the word of the Lord, for Isaac was the son through whom God's promises would be fulfilled. (See Genesis 21:12.) It may have appeared that God had changed His mind, for God was seemingly contradicting Himself. This was a severe test of Abraham's faith and obedience, but Abraham did not complain. He did not even use the word *sacrifice*. Abraham said to the young men that went with them, "Stay here...We [not *I*]) will worship and then we will come back to you" (Gen. 22:5, NIV). He worshiped God; he did not hold on to Isaac. He learned to let loose and surrender everything to God.

How, why, and what was taking place, Abraham did not know; but by faith he obeyed, for Abraham trusted God. The Scripture says Abraham believed God, for in the very act of sacrificing his son, he reckoned that God was able to raise him from the dead. (See Hebrews 11:19.) After Abraham had passed the test, "The angel of the Lord called to him from heaven, and said…'Do not stretch out your hand against the lad…For now I know that you fear God, since you have not withheld your son, your only son, from Me'" (Gen. 22:11–12, NAS). Therefore God said, "I will greatly bless you, and I will greatly multiply your seed as the stars of the heavens…because you have obeyed My voice" (Gen. 22:17–18, NAS).

I began to understand all my previous lessons about Abraham and Isaac and how Abraham had been tested, but I also understood more clearly what had taken place in our lives. Matthew 22:27 says, "You shall love the Lord Your God with all your heart, with all your soul, and with all your mind." For me, this verse meant counting the cost and laying on the altar everything that was precious to me. It meant trusting God no matter how impossible the situation looked. We already had given Simon over to the Lord. That question was settled. All that the Lord was saying to us was, "Do not look at the circumstances!"

I knew the story of Abraham's faith in God. I had heard it many times before. But not until this did I really know what took place, for God never takes a promise away.

> God is not a man, that He should lie…Has He said, and will He not do it? Or has He spoken, and will He not make it good?
>
> —Numbers 23:19, NAS

I realized God's promise to me was still there, and that God will keep His word! All the Lord was asking me was, Would you be willing for Me to reverse the promise if that would glorify Me? The Lord did not take the promise away! He was simply saying, "Don't worry about the promise. Trust Me in this." The Lord does not want us to have faith in faith, or even faith in the promises, as wonderful as that might be. He wants us to have faith in Him!

How can God reverse a promise and yet keep His Word? I leave that up to God. I simply believe and trust the Lord in this. And just as Sarah conceived and bore Abraham a son at the appointed time, so did I believe that Simon's hands and feet would be instantly straightened at the appointed time that God had set.

When the Lord gives us a promise, it might look as if the situation is in reverse, but the one thing we can be sure of is that God will do what He says. I looked up the word *reverse* in *Webster's Dictionary*, and it says a reverse is a "change to the contrary; a change to the opposite in direction, order, sequence, relation, or bearing." It also implies a change in the natural order or position.[21] As it pertains to our faith, it means let go and let God work it out in our lives and in the lives of our loved ones. How the Lord wants to work it out is up to Him. All that God asks from us is to trust Him and to believe God. That is why Abraham was called a friend of God. That is why it says in Genesis 15:6, "And he believed in the LORD, and He accounted it to him for righteousness."

We can put our trust in the Word as long as we understand who is behind that Word—Jesus, who is the Word. We must not lose sight of Him. The Lord tells us not to worry and not to look so much at the promise, but to keep our eyes on Him. After all, He is the author and finisher of your faith! (See Hebrews 12:2.)

21. Webster's American Thesaurus, College Edition (New York: Random House, Inc., 2000), 613.

But my righteous one shall live by faith.

—Hebrews 10:38, NASB

13

OVERCOMING OBSTACLES

Simon, in all these years of waiting on the Lord, developed great qualities in his character that are precious. He developed a lot of patience over the years, and when he sets his mind to do something, he goes after it. I remember one particular day when he excitedly came home from school. "Mom, sit down. I have something to tell you." He sat down across the table from me. His eyes sparkled. "I am going to try out for the basketball team tomorrow! What do you think?" He looked at me with excitement in his eyes. "Do you think I should?" he asked.

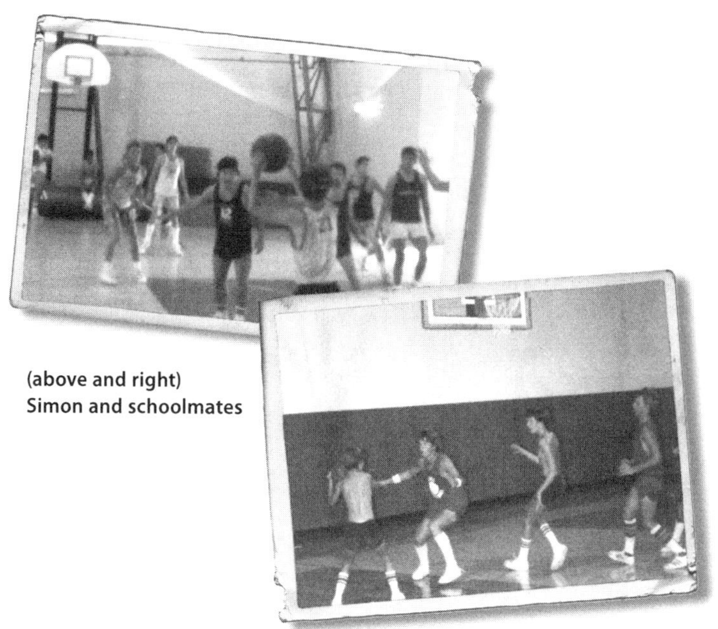

(above and right)
Simon and schoolmates

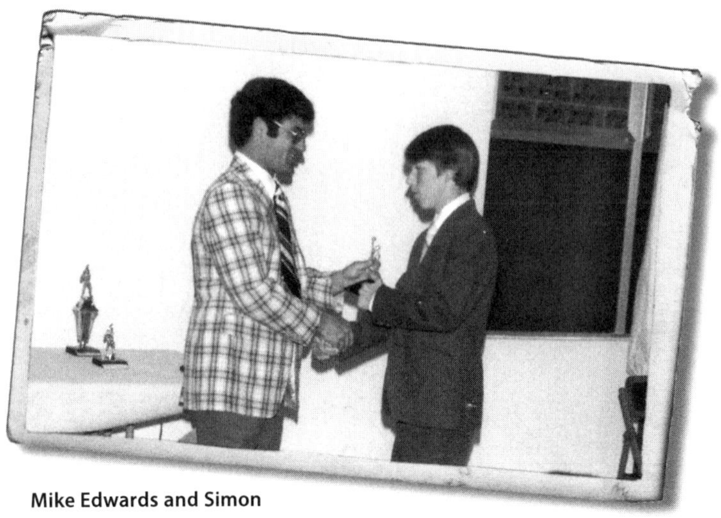

Mike Edwards and Simon

"Yes, go for it, Simon," I said. "If that is what you want to do, then do it." Looking at him, I noticed a wistful gleam in his eyes. "What, Simon? What is it?"

"Oh, Mom, forget it. I can't!"

"Why?" I asked.

"You know Mom, my hands!" A shadow ran across his face. "They are crooked. I can't hold a ball for too long."

"You really want to play, Simon? Well, then, you play and go for it. The Lord will help you, and with God on your side you can do it!" We prayed together that day, asking the Lord to help him. As he got up from the table, he said, "I'll think about it."

Watching him, I knew this was a big decision for him. That evening as we all sat around the dinner table, Simon announced that he was going to try out for the basketball team. And he made the team! And at the end of the basketball season, he had been chosen the most inspirational player of his team! The joy of seeing our son that evening walking down the aisle, clasping his trophy close to him, was another victory! "I can do all things through Christ who strengthens me" (Phil. 4:13).

As I look back over the years, I praise the Lord for all He has done. The Lord restored us all spiritually and gave us the power to face whatever challenges came along. He helped us and gave us the strength to face what we needed. I thank the Lord for everything and in everything. No one knows what life will hold for us; only God knows. He is the master Designer of life when we surrender to Him, for "we know that God causes all things to work together for good…" (Rom. 8:28, NASU). For whom is this true? "…To those who love God, to those who are called according to His purpose" (Rom. 8:28, NASU). How do we know this? Because God has foreknown us. (See Ephesians 1:4.) God has "also predestined [us] to become conformed to the image of His Son…and [those] He predestined, these He also called; and whom He called, these He also justified; and whom He justified, these He also glorified" (Rom. 8:29–30, NAS). Next Paul emphasized, with these words, "What then shall we say to these things. If God is for us, who is against us?" (v. 31, NAS). No one.

While writing this book, I am amazed how the Lord has led us to this moment in our lives. What started out as a possible disaster, God turned around for good.

As a young married mom with four children, I was concerned for our children's welfare, their future, and their walk with the Lord. But in all these years, I learned to trust the Lord in and for everything and to surrender everything to God. This is not only a story of the healing of our son, which is a miracle, but also how the Lord dealt with us as a family an added blessing!

Yes, I believe that God is in everything. In Hannah Whithall Smith's book *The Christian's Secret of a Happy Life*, we read an illustration of a woman who asked if God is in everything. Smith writes that the answer came in a vision:

> She thought she was in a perfectly dark place and that there advanced toward her, from a distance, a body of light which gradually surround and enveloped her and everything around her. As it approached, a voice seemed to say, "This is the presence of God! This is the presence of God!" While surrounded with this presence, all the great and awful things in life seemed to pass before her—fighting armies, wicked men, raging beasts, storms and pestilences, sin and suffering of every kind.
>
> She shrank back at first in terror: but soon she saw that the presence of God so surrounded and enveloped herself and each one of these things that not a lion could reach out its paw, nor a bullet fly through the air, except as the presence of God moved out of the way to permit it.
>
> And she saw that if there were ever so thin a film, as it were, of this glorious Presence between herself and the most terrible violence, not a hair of her head could be ruffled, nor anything touch her, except as the Presence decided to let the evil through. Then all the small and annoying things of life passed before her; and equally she saw that there also she was so enveloped in this presence of God that not a cross look, nor a harsh word, nor petty trial of any kind could affect her, unless God's encircling presence moved out of the way to let it in.[22]

For Hannah Smith and for this woman, the question was forever settled—God is in everything. Joseph understood this principle also. He said to his brothers, "And now do not be grieved or angry with yourselves, because you sold me here;

22. Hannah Whitall Smith, The Christian's Secret of a Happy Life (New York: Ballantine Books, 1986), 115-126.

for God sent me before you to preserve life" (Gen. 45:5, NAS). What a tremendous revelation he had that all his steps were ordered by God. I only have to study the life of Joseph and see the awesome power of God at work to realize that God will, in fact work all things together for the good for those who love God.

Dear brothers, is your life full of difficulties and temptations? Then be happy, for when the way is rough, your patience has a chance to grow, and don't try to squirm out of your problems. For when your patience is finally in full bloom, then you will be ready for anything, strong in character, full and complete.

—James 1:2–4, TLB

14

MIZPAH

ONE DAY I had an appointment with a Jewish doctor who was familiar with Simon's illness. I wanted to share with him what God had done in our lives and how the Lord had healed Simon. So before I went that day, I prayed and asked God to help me, "Let the doctor ask me how Simon is doing, God. Let that be a sign for me to share. He is my doctor, not Simon's, and I do not see him that often." As if in response to my prayer, the doctor inquired, "Mrs. De Vries, how is your son Simon doing?" This provided me with an opportunity to share with him what the Lord had done. I welcomed this opportunity, as I had many times in the past. There were so many non-believers I had shared with in the medical profession, especially doctors.

My doctor was very open when I shared with him, especially the story of Abraham and how he believed the Lord. As I was about to leave, he said, "Mrs. De Vries, will you remember me in your prayers?"

Driving home, I talked to the Lord, pouring out my heart before Him: "God, I do not know what I am doing, sharing what You are doing, even in the medical profession. I see skepticism. 'Scleroderma healed?' Do You know there is no cure for scleroderma? The doctors have asked me this, Lord. Many times I have responded to their question by saying, 'Yes, I know, but God still heals. He did it for my son!'"

The doctor I saw that day was different. He was not a believer, but he did ask for prayer, which was the beginning of seed being planted. I wanted to see things progressing faster, but then I found out that in life everything has its timing. It felt as if I were on a mountaintop, watching the Lord at work. I was only doing what God told me to do. A word here; a word there! It was just that simple, but not fast enough for me. I didn't always see results, but by faith I believed God knew what was going on.

That night I woke up with a word the Lord placed in my heart—*Mizpah*. I did not know what it meant, so I went back to sleep. The next morning, that word did not leave me. Constantly it rang through my mind, until finally I thought, "Let me ask Simen. Maybe he knows what it means." I found him working in the garage, fixing our car. "Simen," I asked, "do you know what the word *Mizpah* means? It has been bothering me the whole morning." My husband started to laugh. "Sure," he said, "Two years ago I did a study on that word." Eager to tell me, he dropped everything and went with me into the house. He opened his Bible to Habakkuk 2:1–4 and as he was reading these verses to me, the Lord quickened them to my heart:

> I will climb my watchtower now and wait to see what answer God will give to my complaint. And the Lord said to me, "Write my answer on a billboard, large and clear, so that anyone can read it at a glance and rush to tell the others. But these things I plan won't happen right away. Slowly, steadily, surely, the time approaches when the vision will be fulfilled. If it seems slow, do not despair, for these things will surely come to pass. Just be patient! They will not be overdue a single day! Note this: Wicked men trust themselves alone [as these Chaldeans do], and fail; but the righteous man trusts in me and lives! (TLB)

He went on to say that the word *Mizpah* means "covenant." He explained that covenants were very important in the Eastern countries. In the time of Abraham there were three types of covenants. The first was the sandal covenant, something commonly used and very important. Two parties would exchange a sandal between one another as a sign of agreement.[23]

The second was a salt covenant, where the parties involved would take some grains of salt out of their bags, which they carried with them, and place them in the bag of the other party.[24] If any of them wanted to get out of the agreement, they simply had to find these same grains of salt that were dropped in their bag and return them. Of course, this was impossible.

The last covenant was called a blood covenant. Here the parties involved would both walk between the slaughtered carcasses of some animals as a token of agreement. If any party did not keep his part of the bargain, he would be slain.

That was the very covenant God-Jehovah made with Abraham. (See Genesis 15:9–23.) He told Abraham to divide specific animals in half and lay each side next to one another. Then He put Abraham in a deep sleep, and in his dream Abraham saw God walk through the split animals. However, Abraham did not have to walk through, signifying that it was God who was going to keep this covenant promise to Abraham. That was when God said, "I will watch between me and thee" (Gen. 31:49, author's paraphrase). I was amazed! I understood.

It is God who watches over His Word to perform it. It is His faithfulness, not our faithfulness; not our faith, but God's faith, for Jesus is the author and finisher of our faith." (See Hebrews 12:2.) A small amount of faith is enough when it is faith placed in a big God.

I began to realize that without God there is nothing we could do. So many Christians have said, "I don't have that kind of faith. How do I get more faith?" All I know is Jesus! If we keep our

---

23. Merrill Unger, New Unger's Bible Dictionary (Chicago, IL: Moody Publishers, 2006), s.v. "sandal covenant."

24. Geoffrey Bromiley, ed., International Standard Bible Encyclopedia (Grand Rapids, MI: Wm. B. Eerdmans Publishing Co., 1979), s.v. "salt covenant."

eyes on Him, we will understand that with God all things are possible.

The disciples asked Jesus this same question after He explained how hard it was for a rich man to be saved. The illustration Jesus used was that of a camel going through the eye of a needle, to which the disciples asked, "Who then can be saved?" (Matt. 19:25). Jesus replied, "With God all things are possible" (v. 26). We serve an all-knowing and loving heavenly Father who knows all of our hurts and disappointments.

Our family saw this vividly demonstrated one Sunday evening after church. After having our usual coffee and snacks, we retired for the evening. As I was about to turn in, I saw Simon sitting alone on the sofa. "Simon," I asked, "what is the matter? Are you not feeling well?"

"Mom," he said, "I had an awful week!"

"Why, Simon?" I asked.

He poured out his heart to me, and as I listened to him I became aware of God's presence with us and knew that God wanted to minister to him in a special way.

"Mom, you keep on telling me that the Lord is going to heal my hands, but when? You and Dad believe it, but I have a difficult time believing. It has taken so long!" Again I told him that God was going to completely straighten out his hands and feet and that the Lord had promised this. Simon, who by this time was a young man of seventeen, was listening and beginning to question many things. "Yes, Mom, you believe, but how can I believe this is so? I want to know for myself."

This is really what all of us have to face, for God is a personal God to each of us. "Simon," I said, "the only way you can find out is to ask God for yourself."

"If the Lord spoke to you, Mom, He can speak to me," was Simon's reply.

"That's right," I said. "How do you want God to speak to you?"

"In the middle of the night," Simon said. "I would like it if God would speak to me in the middle of the night."

"OK," I said. "Let's pray!"

"No, Mom, you pray!"

"No, Simon, you ask the Lord yourself."

With that we held hands and Simon prayed, "Dear God, You told my mom that my hands and feet are going to be straightened. Now I would like to know it for myself. I ask You to reveal it to me also, preferably in the middle of the night. Thank You. In Jesus' name, amen." With that, Simon looked at me and smiled, saying, "We'll see, Mom."

A week went by and nothing happened. I began to wonder, "God, did I tell Simon everything right? It was You, was it not?" Talking to the Lord, my eyes fell on a verse from the book of Jeremiah: "You have seen well, for I am watching over my word to perform it" (Jer. 1:12, RSV). Praising the Lord for His Word, I went about doing my business.

A week later, Simon walked into our bedroom, eyes sparkling. "Mom," he said, "I have something to tell you. Last night as I was asleep I had a dream, and in my dream I was sitting in a church when someone came up to me saying, 'You are being healed. Stand up!' I said to myself, 'Sure,' not really believing. But as I was standing up, I felt the power of God flowing through me like electric currents. Looking at my hands, they were perfectly straight! I said, 'I am healed!'"

What a big God we serve! It never ceases to amaze me how God knows our minute disappointments and how much He wants to minister to and comfort us. Just as the Lord promised, He will watch over His Word to perform it!

And I am sure that God who began the good work within you will keep right on helping you grow in his grace until his task within you is finally finished on that day when Jesus Christ returns.

—Philippians 1:6, TLB

15

THE CALL

AROUND THAT TIME, I heard someone say, "Bloom where you are planted." My husband and I asked the Lord to use us, and we both felt the Lord calling us to the ministry. Exactly where, when, and how we did not know, but we both prepared and went to Bible college by faith.

One day as I was sitting in class, the Lord spoke to my heart, *Television. You will be involved in making TV programs!* Right there in the classroom, the Lord spoke to me. "Television?" I thought. I did not even know how to tape the TV program that we wanted to watch later. But a joy welled up in my heart. "Could this be true? Is this the Lord?" I hoped. By faith we went to school. Simen went in the evening, and when he graduated, I went. The children were all in school by then, so I went in the morning and was home in the afternoon when they came home.

I did not share the Lord's word to me with anyone, thinking, "If this is of the Lord, it will grow." That was a Friday morning, and when Saturday came, I woke up and joy welled up inside me about making television programs! The presence of the Lord stayed with me. Sunday came, and I still pondered this in my heart. Monday morning came and no one was home, but then something happened. There was an overwhelming presence of the Lord in our living room, and I heard myself saying, "All right God, I will find someone perfect for You!" I gave the Lord a lot of reasons why I could not do the job myself.

Then the Lord brought to my attention the story of Mary and Joseph, who were not married when the angel of the Lord appeared to Mary and said that she would be with child.

> And Mary said to the angel, "How can this be, since I am a virgin?" And the angel answered and said to her, "The Holy Spirit will come upon you, and the power of the Most High will overshadow you; and for that reason the holy offspring shall be called the Son of God...For nothing will be impossible with God."
>
> —Luke 1:34–35, 37, nas

Mary's reaction was, "May it be done to me according to your word" (Luke 1:38, NASU). In those days a girl who was pregnant and not married would be stoned to death. But what was Mary's response? "According to your word."

All that was required of me was to be obedient, just as Mary was a long time ago. I knew the presence of the Lord was all around me, and I raised my arms and started to praise and worship the Lord, singing yes to the call of God. I saw the gospel going out all over Europe. How the Lord was going to do this, I did not know, but I believed Him. And so, this promise was fulfilled twenty years later.

When Simen came home that evening, I shared with him what the Lord was going to do. He listened, and a big smile ran across his face. We prayed together and thanked the Lord for calling us to the ministry. What a privilege to work for God. And I might add that I am "confident of this very thing, that He who began a good work in you will perfect it until the day of Christ Jesus" (Phil. 1:6, NAS).

Now to him who is able to do exceeding abundantly beyond all that we ask or think, according to the power that works within us.

—Ephesians 3:20, NASB

EPILOGUE

LOOKING BACK ON our lives, I realize how many prayers have been answered. God, in His infinite wisdom, did not allow some prayers to be answered the way I wanted, while others, He did. But in reality God answered all our prayers, and that is so good!

I have experienced the goodness of God, for He alone is trustworthy, even when we are not. God knows everything about us. When it seems to us that God is nowhere to be found, but then really He is not lost; the problem lies with us. We see only so much, but God knows the beginning from the end:

> O Lord, you have examined my heart and know everything about me. You know when I sit or stand. When far away you know my every thought. You chart the path ahead of me and tell me where to stop and rest. Every moment you know where I am.
>
> —Psalm 139:1–3, TLB

God knew us from before the world began. (See Ephesians 1:4.) God is not surprised about anything. If we surrender our lives to God and let go and let God, anything is possible. When God calls us, He will keep His word: "God is not a man, that he should lie, nor a son of man, that he should change his mind. Does he speak and then not act? Does he promise and not fulfill?" (Num. 23:19, NIV). Of course, God keeps His Word; that goes without saying.

> As the rain and the snow come down from heaven, and do not return to it without watering the earth and making it bud and flourish, so that it yields seed for the sower and bread for the eater, so is my word that goes out from my mouth: It will not return to me empty, but will accomplish what I desire and achieve the purpose for which I sent it.
>
> —Isaiah 55:10–12, NIV

I thank God for everything—the mountaintop experiences and in the valley when I cried out, "God, where are You? What are You doing?" It is there, in that place where we don't like to be, that we grow in the Lord, even though we do not understand until later.

My question to God was, I know You called us into the ministry; but when, where, and how? In answer to one of those all-too-familiar questions, the Lord impressed on us to go to Holland. We boarded a flight from California to Amsterdam, not really knowing what to expect except that as we obeyed God, He would open the door and we would walk right through it. So, by faith, we obeyed.

As we arrived in our hotel room, we decided to call a friend, who invited us for dinner the next day. We rested and prayed, and the next day we met our friends. We got acquainted again, for we had not seen each other in a long time. We had a good time together. Then he said, "There is a meeting in Germany this weekend. Would you like to join us?"

"About what?" we asked.

"It is a conference about how to reach Europe with the gospel via TV and radio. We received an invitation, and maybe you people would like to go, too?"

"We would love to go!" we said. He then gave us the information we needed, and as we left he said, "We'll see you this weekend."

We drove that weekend to Germany, to Schloss Naumburg near Stuttgart in May of 1982. It was the EuroVision Conference in the mountains of Germany, a beautiful place. After we arrived, we settled into our room.

Later in the afternoon we joined the other people, who by then had arrived at the convention. Our eyes were opened; we were not the only people whom God had called to broadcast in Europe. We met people from all over Europe with the same passion and goals of reaching the people in Europe with the good news. We shared, we prayed, and we all worshiped God. There was an exchange of ideas for programs. We listened and took everything in while we heard what was going on in Europe.

The broadcast airwaves in Europe are very much controlled by the government, but today we see rays of hope. The gospel has penetrated Europe and the Middle East by some faithful people who did not give up. The Trinity Broadcasting Network (TBN) is one of the ministries that is greatly used by God to proclaim the gospel, and so have other ministries. As we watched that day, we saw hope, we felt a kinship with the people there from all different kinds of professions, and yet we also had a burden to reach the lost and to spread the gospel.

We had taken some music programs from the U.S. with us, and when we retired to our room, we decided to play it for some of the young people from Europe who were at the conference that day. It was contemporary Christian music. They loved it.

As we watched the video, there was a knock on the door. "May I join you people?" a voice asked. A slender man walked in. We did not know who he was but had seen him at the conference downstairs. He watched the program with us for a while. We started to talk and share, and he introduced himself as Onofrio Miccolis. He produced a program called *100 Percent Living*, aired weekly in Italy and produced in Canada. We were amazed! He was very expressive in his presentation. Everyone was spellbound, for he was a very amicable person, who loved making programs and reaching people with the gospel. We asked a lot of questions that evening.

Then something took place that we did not expect. He turned to us and said, "I want you to meet David Mainse tomorrow. I will arrange it, because I feel we should make a program in Dutch." The next morning we had the privilege to meet with David, president of Crossroads Christian Communications, Inc. of Toronto, Canada. We talked briefly when he said, "Can you come to Toronto and be a guest on our program? I believe the Lord is going to do something. We can also make a pilot program in the Dutch language."

We all felt this was a divine appointment, and we graciously accepted the offer, and Onofrio said, "You can stay at my home!"

"But we have four children," I replied.

"No problem; you are my guests," he answered. That evening we thanked the Lord.

Was this the Lord trying to tell us something? We had a desire to make programs for Holland, yet we were living in the United States. Only God could have orchestrated the solution—a Dutch family living in the U.S.A. meets an Italian television producer at a conference in Germany, only to find that his wife was Dutch also.

As we traveled back to the U.S., we did not really know what all the opportunities would entail, but we did want to follow God and sensed His guidance in our lives. We shared our experience with the rest of our family, and we said, "They all asked us to come in December and make a program. We will see what God is going to do."

Onofrio invited us to stay at his house in Canada, so the whole family went. We were warmly welcomed, and for the first time met his wife and three daughters. As we settled down for the evening, we were expecting the Lord to do something. It was a wonderful time. The next morning we all got acquainted with each other over breakfast. Then the time arrived for serious business. We were going to do a program, but about what? We did not know too much about each other, except that God had put us together for a time like this.

"Well," Onofrio said, "tell me something about yourself. Who are you people?" We all laughed, looking at each other, and said, "Where shall we start?"

"How did you come to know the Lord?" our host began. And as Simen and I shared our story, we felt such a presence of God, knowing this was not an accident and that we were there by divine appointment. "This is God's timing!" we exclaimed.

"Now I know what we are going to do," Onofrio said. "We are doing a story on how you came to know God, how God has healed Simon. And," he added, "we are going to re-enact the whole story!" Then he said, "I knew there was something special about you people." We were all in awe! This was God moving! We were all involved in making our first program. And Simon was asked to give his testimony on *100 Huntley Street*. We had a great time in Canada.

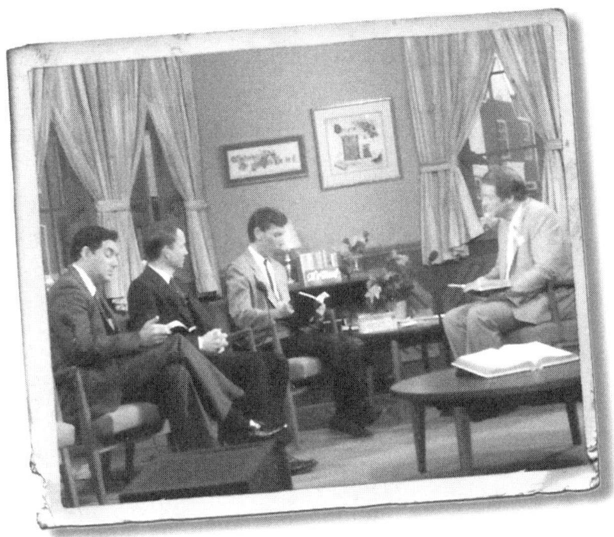

Simon on *100 Huntley Street*

Basically, we shared the story you have read in this book: how God healed our son, how we came to know God, and that all things work together for good for those who love God. We made many more programs after the first. Our first program was shown on the New World Channel, TV 5, a French satellite. By faith we made the first programs, believing that God would open the door—and He did.

We rented the truck from Onofrio that he used to make his programs for Italy. It was stationed in Italy. The truck was equipped with cameras and everything needed to make programs. There were about ten people on the truck. They came from Italy, Sweden, Norway, Holland, and Canada. We stayed at the hotel for about four weeks, made fifty programs, and had a marvelous time doing this. God provided the money, and we learned a lot. Eventually we produced our own programs.

Today, our children, all grown with families of their own, are still involved in the ministry. Jacqueline is a guest on the program and teaches from time to time. Simon is sometimes involved doing camera work, Michael offers his financial support, and Yvonne helps doing the camera when we need her. We are blessed.

We always took our children with us overseas to Europe and exposed them to the ministry. The whole family was involved in our first program, *I Believe in Miracles*. I marvel at what the Lord has done. We could not have imagined this. That is what is meant by the scripture that says, "No mere man has ever seen, heard, or even imagined what wonderful things God has ready for those who love the Lord" (1 Cor. 2:9, TLB).

God is not looking for perfect vessels, but He is looking for yielded vessels. You don't have to be perfect, for no one is. But if you put what you have in God's hands, something good is going to happen.

Currently, we still broadcast all over Europe over TBN and on the local cable in Amsterdam, Salto TV. God is so faithful!

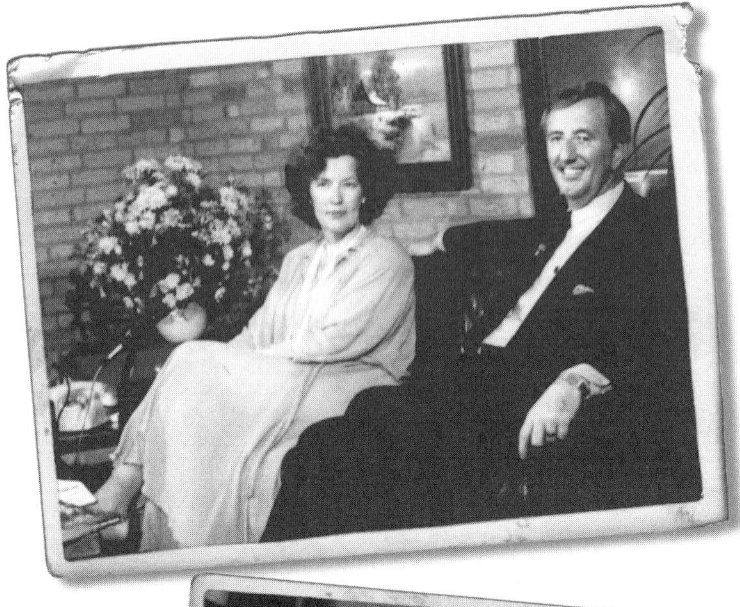

(above) Attie and Simen

(R) Simon

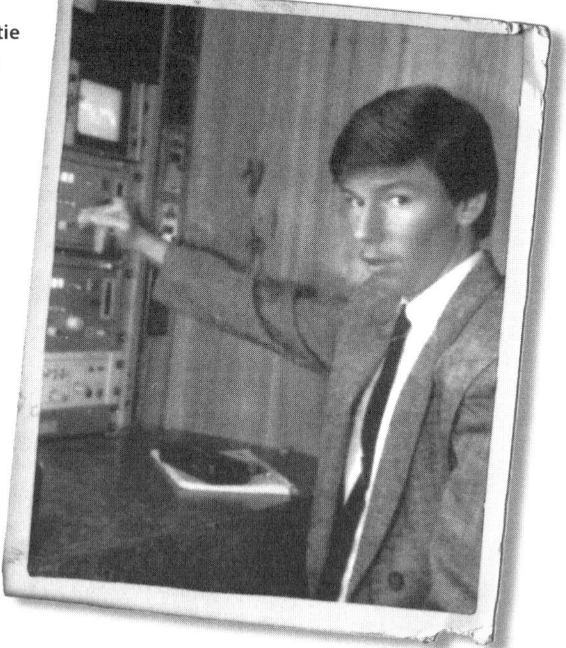

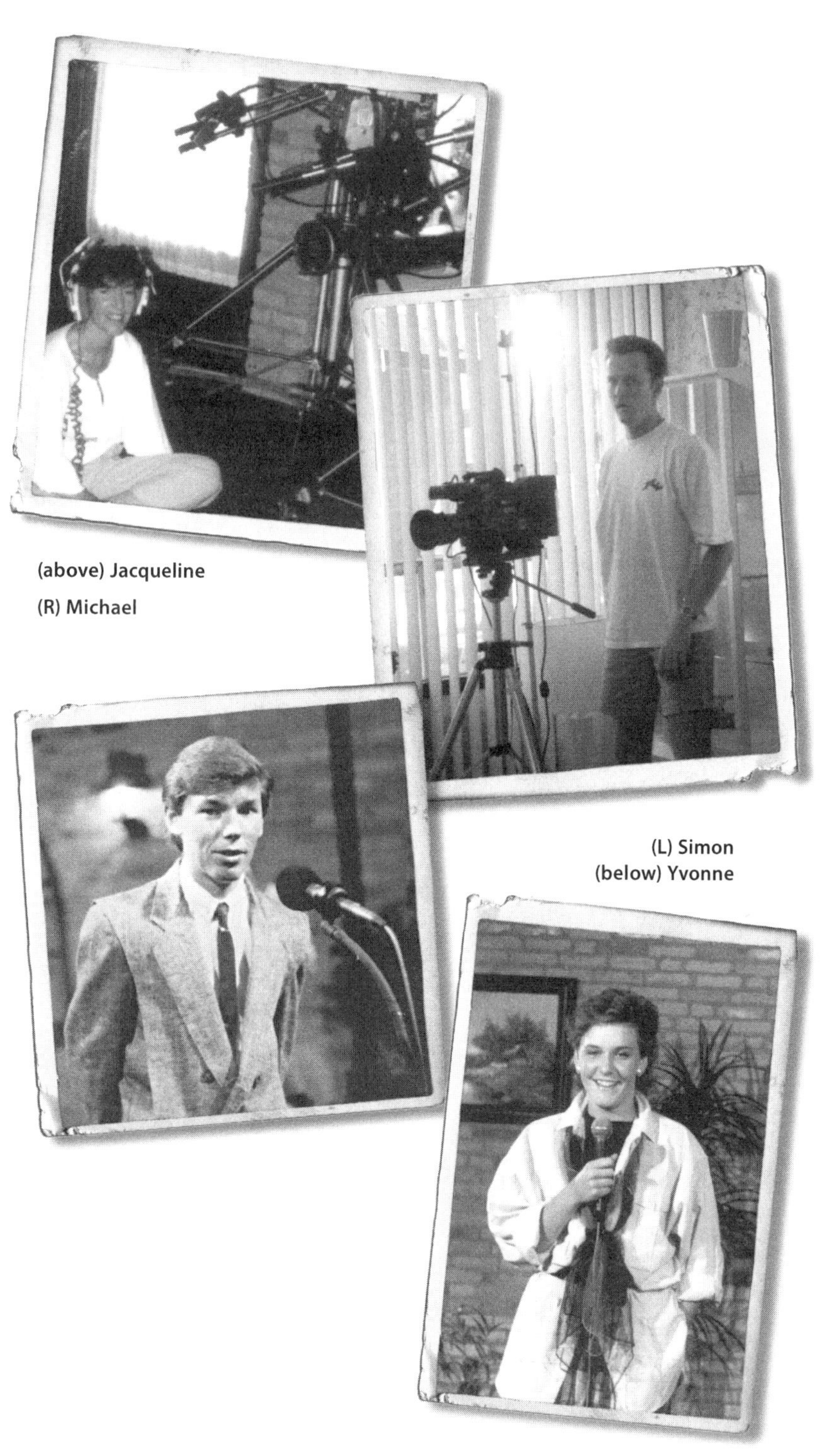

(above) Jacqueline

(R) Michael

(L) Simon

(below) Yvonne

If you have been touched by this story and do not know the Lord, but you want to, then pray this simple prayer and ask Jesus to come into your heart. The Lord will help you.

> *Dear God, I need You. I have made a mess of my life. I want to know You. I believe that You sent Your Son Jesus to die for my sins on the cross. I believe that Your blood was shed on the cross for me. Please forgive me of my sins and come into my heart. In Jesus' name, amen!*

If you prayed this prayer, we would like to hear from you. You can contact us at attiedv@aol.com, or visit us at our Web sites: www.wonderenvandaag.org, or www.attiedevries.com.